Better Patient Feedback, Better Healthcare

Other books from M&K include

The Primary Care Guide to Mental Health
ISBN: 9781905539109

The Clinician's Guide to Chronic Disease Management for Long-Term Conditions:
A cognitive-behavioural approach
ISBN: 9781905539154

Therapy Skills for Healthcare: An introduction to brief psychological techniques
ISBN: 9781905539581

Perinatal Mental Health: A clinical guide
ISBN: 9781905539499

Preventing and Reducing Aggression & Violence in Health and Social Care:
A holistic approach
ISBN: 9781905539574

My Health, My Faith, My Culture: A guide for healthcare practitioners
ISBN: 9781905539802

Identification and Treatment of Alcohol Dependency
ISBN: 9781905539161

Nurses and Their Patients: Informing practice through psychodynamic insights
ISBN: 9781905539314

Better Patient Feedback, Better Healthcare

Dr Taher Mahmud

Foreword by Professor Sir Graeme Catto

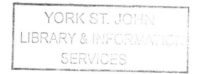

Better Patient Feedback, Better Healthcare
Dr Taher Mahmud

ISBN: 978-1-905-539-24-6

First published 2012

British Library Cataloguing in Publication Data
A catalogue record for this book is available from the British Library

Notice

Clinical practice and medical knowledge constantly evolve. Standard safety precautions must be followed, but, as knowledge is broadened by research, changes in practice, treatment and drug therapy may become necessary or appropriate. Readers must check the most current product information provided by the manufacturer of each drug to be administered and verify the dosages and correct administration, as well as contraindications. It is the responsibility of the practitioner, utilising the experience and knowledge of the patient, to determine dosages and the best treatment for each individual patient. Any brands mentioned in this book are as examples only and are not endorsed by the publisher. Neither the publisher nor the authors assume any liability for any injury and/or damage to persons or property arising from this publication.

To contact M&K Publishing write to:
M&K Update Ltd · The Old Bakery · St. John's Street
Keswick · Cumbria CA12 5AS
Tel: 01768 773030 · Fax: 01768 781099
publishing@mkupdate.co.uk
www.mkupdate.co.uk

Designed and typeset by Mary Blood
Printed in England by H&H Reeds, Penrith

Contents

To my patients and mentors

Foreword

This small volume fulfils a real need. Of course, much has already been written about improving patient care and some improvements have undoubtedly been achieved. However, this book provides practical guidance on how best to evaluate patients' views on the care they have received and how to implement the necessary improvements.

Taher Mahmud and the other contributors have considerable experience of promoting changes in important areas of clinical practice, and their views will undoubtedly prove influential in helping to secure further improvements in patient care.

Over the centuries, good clinicians have always modified their practices to meet the needs of their patients; it is only comparatively recently that the increasing complexity of modern medicine and its organisation has made such flexibility more difficult to attain.

All clinicians accept that care must be patient-centred, but putting that concept into practice often proves difficult. If care is to be truly patient-led, we shall all have to reassess how we determine the views and needs of our patients, and then find new ways to evaluate the extent to which our practice meets their legitimate expectations.

The information provided in this lucid and succinct book shows the patient involvement perspectives. I hope this small volume will encourage you to pilot patient feedback as outlined in this book, and then to contribute to collective efforts regarding improving patient experiences and their clinical outcomes.

Professor Sir Graeme Catto

Professor Sir Graeme Catto is former President of the General Medical Council, and Emeritus Professor of Medicine at the University of Aberdeen. He has also served as Chief Scientist for the NHS in Scotland and Vice-Principal at King's College London, Dean of King's College, Guy's and St Thomas' Hospitals' Medical and Dental Schools, and Pro-Vice Chancellor, University of London.

About the author

Taher Mahmud commenced his medical training as a student at King's College London and trained in General Medicine at King's College Hospital and St Thomas' Hospital, before specialising in Rheumatology at King's College Hospital, St Thomas' and Guy's Hospitals.

Taher has worked in a number of teaching and district general hospitals; he has also served as an Honorary Consultant at the Royal National Hospital for Rheumatic Diseases in Bath. Taher now has a Rheumatology practice at Tunbridge Wells Hospital at Pembury. He is also Lead for Osteoporosis and former Lead for Clinical Governance in Acute Medicine and Clinical Audit. He set up the Arthritis Centre (www.arthritiscentre.org), with the aim of providing early multidisciplinary care for people with arthritis.

Taher remains passionate about the quality of clinical care delivered to patients. His ongoing studies and improvements in this area have undoubtedly contributed to his success in achieving a Clinical Excellence Award. In addition, he has received the NHS Innovations South East Inventor Award for his work on systematic, continuous, real-time patient feedback over the long term.

Taher also founded the Centre for Patient Involvement (www.patientinvolvement. org), which provides a forum in which to share the best practical approaches to patient feedback and patient care.

Contributors

The content of this small volume is based in part on the contributions to two conferences organised to look at patient involvement at the Royal Society of Medicine and King's Fund.

This book features input on patient perspective from Suzie Hughes (Chair of the Patient and Carer Network at the Royal College of Physicians), Federico Moscogiuri (Head of Policy and Campaigns at Arthritis Care) and Jenny Snell, (Government Affairs Manager at National Rheumatoid Arthritis Society).

The perspective of a large acute hospital group is from Glenn Douglas, CEO, Maidstone and Tunbridge Wells NHS Trust.

The perspective of a medical regulator is from Mr Paul Buckley, while Director of Education and Revalidation, and Una Lane, Director of Continued Practice and Revalidation at the General Medical Council.

The national healthcare view and vision setting is from the Department of Health, Sir David Nicholson CBE, NHS Chief Executive, and Sir Donald Irvine, former GMC President and Chair of the Picker Foundation.

Introduction

This book attempts to capture the output from several conferences and includes a variety of perspectives on patient feedback and patient involvement. The patient perspective is provided by: Suzie Hughes, Chair of the Patient and Carer Network at the Royal College of Physicians; Federico Moscogiuri, Head of Policy and Campaigns at Arthritis Care; and Jenny Snell, Government Affairs Manager at the National Rheumatoid Arthritis Society. The perspective of a large acute hospital group comes from Glenn Douglas, Chief Executive, Maidstone and Tunbridge Wells NHS Trust.

The perspective of medical regulators is provided by: Mr Paul Buckley, while Director of Education and Revalidation; and Una Lane, Director of Continued Practice and Revalidation at the General Medical Council.

The clinician's perspective comes from Taher Mahmud, who has a long-standing interest in the practical issues surrounding patient feedback in a range of clinical settings.

The national healthcare view and vision setting from the Department of Health is offered by: Sir David Nicholson CBE, NHS Chief Executive; and Sir Donald Irvine, former General Medical Council President and now Chair of the Picker Institute Europe.

It is very important to understand the link between patient outcomes and clinician–patient interactions. Building better communication through systematic patient feedback could enable many healthcare workers to improve patient care and team effectiveness. To this end, this book explores ideas and methodologies related to patient feedback and care, and outlines effective methods of measuring, analysing and enhancing feedback.

In this volume, you will find a variety of useful opinions, strategies and techniques. We also summarise current views on patient involvement from the National Association of Rheumatoid Arthritis and Arthritis Care, the King's Fund, the General Medical Council and the Royal College of Physicians, as well as the Department of Health. The presentations of these organisations at the patient involvement conferences in 2009 and 2010 (at the Royal Society of Medicine and King's Fund) are accessible via the www.patientinvolvement.org website and were the catalysts for this publication.

The book offers helpful information that we hope will enable clinicians and patients to discuss the best ways to put feedback approaches and systems in place. Ultimately, we aim to contribute to a move towards real-time (immediate) patient feedback systems in all healthcare settings. The potential benefits of these feedback systems include improved patient care, improved patient–clinician communication and more effective team self-review. In the long term, such approaches can lead to continual small improvements that cumulatively add up to major transformation in healthcare systems.

Despite the implementation of various government policies, until recently patient involvement and patient feedback have not had a very high profile in clinical practice. There has been no tradition of systematically seeking and tracking patient feedback over time – let alone using that feedback to continually review and improve services.

So why do we believe it is so vital to gather patient feedback? One reason is the now widely observed fact that only 50 % of patients with long-term conditions take their treatments as recommended by doctors. In other words, only half our patients make use of our advice and benefit fully from the treatments we have offered them! Realising this makes clinicians very uncomfortable and gives us a strong desire to improve our effectiveness as healthcare professionals. Long-term conditions take up 80 % of healthcare budgets so improving the effectiveness of treatment has major financial implications as well as obvious importance for quality of patient care. For further information on this, visit: **www.youtube.com/user/AchievingPI09?feature = watch**

We also find that the patient feedback process can help patients to feel more valued and understood. This creates an improved rapport between patient and clinician, which benefits both. Better outcomes for patients will enable them to remain active and productive for longer and will in fact produce cost savings. At a time when health costs are escalating, with a demand for increasingly complex and expensive treatments, patient feedback has an important role in addressing patient need and improving treatment adherence.

In clinical settings where staff members are busy dealing with many different screening and checking systems, employing the techniques in this book may seem like adding yet another burden to an already heavy workload. However, we have found that implementing a good patient feedback system actually helps to *streamline* services.

Furthermore, patient feedback will increasingly be used by NHS healthcare commissioners for reimbursement purposes. This is being proposed in the UK and is already happening in the Medicaid system employed in the USA.

Acknowledgements

I am grateful to all my patients and colleagues who have shared their insights and helped with the patient feedback pilot schemes. I am also grateful to the teams I have worked with over the years and to Ali Afzal (junior doctor), Louise Moss (medical secretary) and Hilary Joy (hospital manager) for producing the very first patient questionnaire.

I would particularly like to thank Suzie Hughes, Federico Moscogiuri, Jenny Snell, Glenn Douglas, Paul Buckley, Una Lane, Sir David Nicholson and Sir Donald Irvine for their contributions; without their generous input this book would not have been possible.

I appreciate the mentoring I constantly receive from my patients in improving clinical interaction, and I am thankful to my family for their encouragement.

Finally, I am indebted to Professor Sir Graeme Catto, Professor Elisabeth Paice and Professor Bernard Crump for their kind mentorship over the years.

Chapter 1

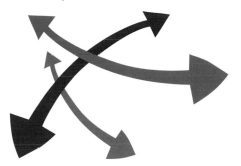

Fundamentals of Patient Feedback

When establishing or revising patient feedback procedures, it is vital to set guidelines across the board. Consistency is the key to gaining optimum benefits from a comprehensive patient feedback system. Without this formalised, consistent structure, results may be inaccurate or incomplete and will not deliver continuing benefits to patients.

At the patient involvement conferences held in 2009 and 2010, the case for better patient involvement was well made by Suzie Hughes (Chair of the Patient and Carer Network at the Royal College of Physicians), Federico Moscogiuri (Head of Policy and Campaigns at Arthritis Care) and Jenny Snell (Government Affairs Manager at the National Rheumatoid Arthritis Society). Having worked with a diverse group of patients, they all found that patients were very pleased to be more involved in their own care. They argued that participating in feedback can form the basis of a patient–clinician partnership, with patients setting the direction and making treatment choices with the guidance of the clinical team.

Golden rules of setting up patient feedback systems

It is possible for each team in a healthcare service to have its own feedback system. However, better value will be gained by having the same system of patient feedback in use across a whole organisation. Otherwise inconsistent feedback practices will result in uneven and unrealistic statistics, which are not useful for analytical and planning purposes. Therefore, after deciding upon the right patient feedback system for your facility or department, you should make sure that the same feedback guidelines are followed in every case. In most scenarios, setting up a 'chain of command' (to be certain that new or revamped patient feedback rules and regulations are being followed) will be a smart move and a good starting point.

If you are in charge of setting up or revamping a patient feedback system, you should start by making a project plan as follows:

1. Establish the case for a new or revised patient feedback system.
2. Gain an understanding of the current situation (e.g. any feedback/complaints system that is already in use).
3. Identify any recurring issues (e.g. do many complaints involve poor clinical care and/or poor communication?).
4. Build local and organisational support for the new system.
5. Gather the resources and team members needed to carry out the project.
6. Appoint a project manager and ensure that they have a project plan.
7. Carry out pilots and share the findings; encourage wider adoption of the feedback system and ongoing improvement.
8. For the system to become properly embedded, you will need the senior executive, clinicians, clerks, nurses and patients to 'buy in' (commit) to it.
9. It is important to make a start as soon as possible; sometimes projects can be unduly delayed and all momentum lost.

Since soliciting feedback from patients is a part of patient–clinician interaction, it's crucial that the tone and attitude of all staff is positive, compassionate and professional. Positive interactions come from positive attitudes. These interactions will usually lead to more detailed responses, which is exactly what is needed to get valuable feedback.

Barriers to implementation

As with any new initiative, there will be barriers that stand in the way of implementing an effective new or revamped patient feedback system. In our experience, individual healthcare workers and institutions often have a genuine fear of inviting continuous feedback from patients. This fear is misplaced. Patients are usually very generous with their feedback. They can offer valuable insights and their complaints and concerns are usually well founded.

Frequently expressed concerns about instituting organisation-wide feedback systems may include: adding to patient waiting times, budget pressures, shortage of resources required for staff training, and pressures caused by understaffing.

Although such barriers will always surface, they do not necessarily have to result in the failure or diminished success of your system, provided your project has been well planned and is well supported. You will have to become skilled at recognising and dealing with the underlying motives behind such obstructions.

By streamlining your patient feedback system to reflect the number of staff you have available, as well as typical waiting times and other common barriers, you can create a system that is tailored to the specific needs of your clinical teams and patients. In time, it may be possible to expand your new system to other clinical teams and other aspects of your service.

It's important to remember that better patient feedback will in the future be reflected in the tariff your unit can expect to receive from the service provider. From the clinician's perspective, better patient engagement can lead to better service delivery and a greater likelihood that patients will adhere to prescribed treatments. Therefore, the short-term expenditure necessary to roll out a new system of patient feedback will eventually be offset or balanced by long-term savings at the operational level – not to mention improved clinical outcomes and eventual reduced health spend.

Barriers should be reduced and resolved where possible, but they should never be an excuse to refrain from carrying out patient feedback and improving clinical service. After all, the relationship between patient feedback and the patient's overall progress is often intertwined. The more feedback patients give, the more likely it is that they will reveal issues that might impact on their adherence to treatment. For example, in our clinics we hear patients sharing the fact that they are not taking some of the treatments they have been recommended by another clinic. They also say that they tell that team that they are taking their treatment when they are not!

As teams gain confidence in routinely soliciting patient feedback, they will become more comfortable about receiving feedback. In our pilots in different clinical settings (both hospital and primary care), implementing systems of feedback has resulted in teams reporting a sense of empowerment – both healthcare staff and patients feel more listened to. The key driver for patient engagement in feedback is demonstrating action based on the feedback received. In other words, if patients see changes being made in response to their comments, to better serve their needs, they will be encouraged to share more insights.

Enhanced patient feedback has become an important new facet of intake, treatment and follow-up for patients, as shown by the following examples.

Innovative leadership

Arthritis Care (AC) is the United Kingdom's largest supporter of people living with arthritis. Founded in 1947 (one year before the NHS was established), this worthwhile and innovative organisation has always pioneered self-management for people with arthritis. The agency has a user-led approach, and the majority of AC employees are arthritis patients themselves. For example, Neil Bettridge, CEO of Arthritis Care, developed rheumatoid arthritis at the age of three, and he has come to believe that self-management is the key to successful treatment. Frederico Mascogiuri is Head of Policy and Campaigns at Arthritis Care, and he shared (at the Royal Society of Medicine Conference in 2009) his experiences of improving patient knowledge and self-management. He also suggested improvements to the complex healthcare system *from a patient's perspective*.

> The AC work shows there is an increasing emphasis on patient and public involvement, especially since the Darzi Review [a report detailing a ten-year plan for the NHS, written by Lord Darzi while he was Health Minister] was published in 2008. This world-class NHS Commission now requires commissioners to engage more directly with service users. The NHS constitution states the need for patients to be given the right [and] the means to be involved, and the ability to express their opinions.
>
> The NHS is re-orientating itself to deliver high-quality and inclusive services across the board, based on patient experience; these means will generally meet the needs of people concerned ... the concept is based on a growing recognition that patients are in the best position to know how their conditions and treatments affect them and what they need from healthcare providers in the health service.
>
> Overall, there are encouraging signs for a more patient-centred health service. However, getting there will be (and has been) a difficult undertaking. At present, the level of clinical engagement is '*very patchy*' at best.
>
> World-class commissioning shows us that engagement is currently far from what its name might suggest. On average, 1.6 out of 4 was scored in overall satisfaction from Primary Care Trusts. A recent Healthcare Commission report showed that people felt they didn't have enough say regarding services, which directly affected them. Clearly, the reality is struggling to live up to the rhetoric – there is an obvious need for better, more proactive involvement of patients and service users.

Involvement or engagement?

According to Frederico Mascogiuri at Arthritis Care, the difference between involvement and engagement may occasionally be misunderstood. As far as Arthritis Care is concerned, *involvement* is the key to improving services for patients. Involvement is the participative element, and it is what every healthcare team needs to aim for. In contrast, *engagement* merely refers to making contact, which is important – but not as potentially useful as involvement.

Arthritis Care has introduced a programme that involves users as experts. This programme consists of a series of courses, which were rolled out from 2007 to 2009. The courses were aimed at empowering people with arthritis and other musculoskeletal conditions, so that they would feel that they were actively involved in the design and delivery of services that affected them. Courses were two-day residentials, and a total of five were completed – three in 2007 and two in June/July 2009. Arthritis Care's devotion to involvement (as opposed to engagement) is a worthy model for more intense and proactive patient feedback. Devising a system in which individual patients feel more involved in their treatment can be the key to more successful treatment. There are various ways to foster a closer connection between patients, clinicians and other medical staff. For example, workshops, meetings, one-on-one (feedback-based) appointments and surveys could be combined.

Getting started

Since the first priority is to establish a patient-led system, the patient must be the focus of planning right from the start. It is crucial to formulate patient feedback guidelines with sensitivity and tact, observing political correctness and etiquette. Here is a suggested approach to setting up a patient–clinician user group, which can provide a useful forum for discussing patient concerns and service development plans.

The most direct method is to appoint patient representatives and clinical and managerial team members who meet at regular intervals (between two and four times a year). These meetings are probably best led and organised by a patient within the relevant department. The meetings need not be more than an hour long. Provided that they are well structured, they can be very productive.

Setting up a patient–clinical team forum

There must be a defined purpose to any successful interaction, so the first step in creating successful interaction between clinicians/managerial staff and patients is setting an agenda (just as there is almost always a defined agenda at any useful business meeting). You need to think about the goal of the interaction, and use that end point as a basis for your agenda. For example, if the patient is seeking to change service delivery, the agenda should be focused on bringing patient and clinician closer together through better approaches on the different challenges and needs.

The agenda should focus conversation towards the goal of establishing better communication and improvements in the service, and the chair should ensure that this remains the focus. As at any formal business meeting, notes (or minutes) should be taken to record the agenda, outcomes and actions; and these notes should be circulated after the meeting.

Optimising clinical consultation

There are a few aspects to be mindful of during patient consultations that will improve patient feedback.

Communicate properly

Communicating effectively during a consultation requires good eye contact, as well as the right tone of voice, body language and manner. Some patients may be uneasy in the presence of certain clinicians, who may seem too cool in manner, or too intellectual or business-like to chat with in a more casual way. Breaking down the barriers between patient and clinician is a tricky business, as there must naturally be some division here.

The best way to approach the issue of better communication is through steady, friendly eye contact, a warmer-than-typical manner, and the use of clear, easy-to-understand language. For example, complex medical terms, ideas and concepts should be explained in layman's terms so that patients from a wide range of backgrounds and educational levels can easily understand them.

Agree on a treatment plan

The patient and clinician should together devise and agree a course of treatment. Although clinicians will always lead care by virtue of their education, skills, credentials and experience, patients should be made to feel that they too have a say in the direction of treatment. If options are available, the patient should be given all the information they need to make a choice about what is best, and they should be supported in their decision-making.

These sorts of meetings also support better self-care by patients. Once patients begin to enjoy more intense communication with their clinicians, as well as greater input into decision-making regarding treatment options, they tend to become more adept at self-care and coping with their condition. The sense of empowerment that comes from better patient feedback and more involvement with clinicians can create a ripple effect that significantly improves the life of a patient and the way they view their health problem.

Of course, the personalities of patients and clinicians will always have an impact on the relative success of meetings and other patient feedback situations. Some relationships will be easier or more relaxed than others. However, regardless of personalities, clinicians involved in our pilots have found the feedback process relatively easy and say that it has had considerable value for them, both individually and for the service as a whole.

In order to make gains across the board, clinicians must take action based on the findings from patient feedback wherever possible, as quickly as possible. Even the most difficult or reticent patient may share worthwhile information about treatment experiences and health issues. In fact, these types of patients, who are more inclined to share criticisms of the healthcare system, often have much to contribute.

In our experience, complaints are the most valuable feedback of all. For decades, entrepreneurs and chief executives of commercial companies have recognised the value of complaints and criticisms, because they can be addressed and changes can be made accordingly. Getting vital feedback can therefore lay the foundation of a refined healthcare delivery system that truly meets the requirements of those who need it most.

Other feedback-gathering options

The team (or individual clinician) can review their interactions with patients immediately after the consultation. This is a powerful approach to determining their effectiveness and can be done 'in real time'.

Patients can also undergo a qualitative interview with a researcher to gain understanding of their experience and care. Although this approach can give considerable insight, it can be time-consuming and costly to carry out.

Therefore, it's often useful to use a variety of different approaches. For example, patient feedback surveys are an excellent way to ask direct questions and track responses (and any patterns that may emerge from those responses). By improving your meetings with patients, and consistently distributing patient feedback forms according to an organised schedule, you can cover all the bases.

Questionnaire tips

Here are some points that you should bear in mind when designing a patient feedback survey:

1 Keep it simple

For some people, filling out patient feedback forms may feel like a chore, and these patients will probably be daunted by anything that seems too complicated. While a minority of patients will want to share their thoughts and impressions in more detail, most patients will prefer to rate their experiences on a number or letter scale, or simply give a 'Yes' or 'No' answer to a specific question.

Therefore, simple forms that offer plenty of extra space for any additional comments are usually the best bet. One page should be sufficient – some clinics or hospitals will have longer forms, including two-sided forms. These may be fine, but in general simpler and shorter really is better. Often, a trial and error period may be necessary before it becomes clear exactly which types of forms are best for a specific clinic or department.

2 Consider the patient

Remember that certain patients may have difficulty writing and that these people may prefer to avoid writing whenever possible. Patients with arthritis, essential tremors,

Parkinson's disease and other similar ailments may need assistance to complete their forms. If writing is a problem for them, every effort should be made to assist them or find an alternative method of getting feedback.

Always consider the barriers created by a patient's specific health problem before offering them a form to fill in. In some cases, it will be more sensitive to get the feedback in another way, such as having a conversation and recording the patient's answers. However, patient feedback forms do give patients a greater sense of privacy and anonymity. They will sometimes reveal more of their true thoughts and emotions than they would in a face-to-face interaction, and this can result in very honest assessments of care.

3 Choose your questions carefully

The way your patients rank their experiences at your healthcare facility can be very illuminating, especially when your surveys are analysed across the board. Therefore, you should carefully consider which aspects of patient experience you want to question patients about. From waiting times to the politeness of receptionists to the comfort of your waiting rooms – make sure you ask the right questions in order to get the information you really need.

Since asking too many questions is to be avoided, it's important to streamline your form to get the data you really need to make a difference. For example, if patients are reporting poor satisfaction with your waiting room, there may be various reasons why they don't feel comfortable there. From temperatures that are too high or too low to the wrong type of seating, to old magazines or too much ambient noise – there can be many different variables. For this reason, asking a couple of additional questions about *why* patients are dissatisfied may enable you to rectify specific problems and improve the whole patient experience.

Patient feedback on the Internet

Nowadays, some healthcare providers offer patients an alternative way to comment on services, whether anonymously or not. Since many facilities now have websites with comment areas, it's important to know how to deal with this type of feedback and to be aware of the pros and cons.

The advantages of getting patient feedback online are the immediacy and convenience of this form of communication. Patients can complete a questionnaire either in the clinic or afterwards – and the location can be tracked, using identification of clinics and clinicians. The feedback can compiled/collated automatically – there are several software programs available, including ones by Dr Foster (www.drfosterhealth.co.uk/). The clinical team and hospital administrators can access the information here, and our advice would be to share feedback results with patients. For an example of how to show such information, see **www.arthritiscentre.org/patient-feedback/feedback-1/**

Patients can comment directly on their clinic experience on the institution's website or at a general feedback website such as Patient Opinion (**www.patientopinion.org.uk/**) or iwantgreatcare (**www.iwantgreatcare.org/**).

The Internet is a good way of letting patients know about the services you provide for them, simply by adding website URL address information to pamphlets, forms, letters and other paperwork. A website can also offer a way of updating patients about the services offered and keeping them in contact with the department.

The downside to having patient feedback on a website is the amount of time it can take to oversee the service. Also, anonymous comments may be very honest, occasionally to the point of rudeness or profanity. There is also a risk that a disgruntled or disturbed patient or other individual may unfairly smear a facility's reputation. These problems can be best avoided by using an external agency to record the comments, from validated individuals only (their personal details will not be shared with the institution).

In other cases, patients will be complimentary or leave comments that are a mixture of good and bad. Since a healthcare facility's website is an online portal that also acts as a virtual advertisement or business profile, negative or strange comments may harm a clinic's (or clinician's) reputation. If you wish to address anonymous comments on your website, this sort of interaction must be carefully handled.

Here are some tips on soliciting and responding to feedback that is sent to your website.

1 Moderate comments

When setting up your online patient feedback system, you should choose to moderate comments. Adding this feature will allow you to see comments before anyone else does, and you will also be able to decide whether or not comments should be posted to your website. While some patients may be displeased to see that their comments have been rejected, this feature provides a layer of protection designed to shield your website from spam comments, overly malicious remarks, and so on. Once you've posted a moderated comment that others can also see on your website, you should respond under a neutral username.

2 Respond under a general username

The general advice would be that clinicians should not respond to clinical questions posted on the website. If individual clinicians wish to do this, they can do so personally on their own websites and blogs. Generally, it is not possible to provide reliable clinical advice without having seen the patient previously.

3 Set boundaries

Patients should always be aware that any advice or information on the website is no substitute for a proper diagnosis or treatment. All individuals wishing to seek medical advice should see a qualified physician or clinician.

Making use of social networks

Once you have established a framework for your online presence, you may wish to include Twitter, Facebook and MySpace. (MySpace has become less popular, but is still used by some people.) These social networks can offer a great platform for providing useful tips on health and well-being.

These days almost every business (profit or non-profit) has a social networking presence, and yours should be no exception. The rules of social networking are similar to the rules of commenting at your website; however, social networking may require more outreach from you or your team.

In order to get the best results, you will need to connect with people by adding them as 'friends' (as with Facebook) or 'following' them on Twitter. Including your account details in the different communications will increase web traffic and will provide your online visitors with tweets about your clinical services, facilities, and any special events or wellness tips. This sort of social networking initiative can add value to the patient experience by giving patients another way to connect with you outside your facility.

Before dismissing this aspect of community outreach, bear in mind that many people nowadays *do* look to health websites for information about self-care, symptoms, home remedies and medical advice. In fact, it's been proved that almost 50 per cent of the population refers to health websites when they are researching a health issue. Therefore, developing an online presence can be very beneficial when it comes to improving patient feedback – and in order to assist the online patient community.

To add even more value, you can link to articles about self-care, diet, exercise and other helpful advice. Adding photos of your facility can also be a great way to promote the activities of your institution and bond with patients online. Usually, you can manage social media in about 15 minutes per day; in fact, there are services, such as Tweetdeck and SocialOomph, which allow you to streamline your updates and track other's accounts. It's also possible to schedule plenty of updates in advance to save yourself the trouble of logging in daily. Of course, no patient information should ever be put online; after all, there is no real data security and everything is public.

Now that we've discussed some options for fact gathering and staying in touch with patients, let's consider other elements that are relevant to enhanced patient feedback.

Reducing waiting times

Most clinicians and healthcare professionals already know that waiting times have a pronounced effect on patient satisfaction. This book is focused on teaching self-care and improving patient health through better feedback systems; however, the issue of waiting times will always be important. It seems counter-productive to channel a lot of energy and effort into improving communication with your patients if they are always going to be irritated and frustrated when they meet you after a very long stay in a waiting room.

Therefore, it is well worth addressing the issue of clinic waiting times. Not surprisingly, studies show that clinics with shorter waiting times demonstrate higher patient satisfaction averages. Obviously, the shorter the time that patients have to wait, the happier they are. However, their main priority is to have all clinical issues dealt with. In fact, some patients apparently view longer waiting times as a sign that the clinician is particularly thorough!

In the experience of my own NHS team, by constantly reviewing the running of the clinic and making small changes, we were able to bring down the waiting times, even though we increased the number of patients seen per hour from three to four. The patients expressed greater satisfaction too. This has led us to think that it is not necessarily the length of time that patients spend with the clinician but the quality of the communication that determines patient satisfaction and the overall effectiveness of the team. In reviewing the effectiveness of use of health resources and staff/clinic times it is worth looking at the possibility of changing some work practices.

1 Look at consultation patterns

Firstly, many consultations may not be strictly necessary or appropriate. For example, certain question-and-answer sessions between clinicians and patients may not require face-to-face meetings. If there are ways to reduce the total number of consultations through phone calls, email or other methods that don't interfere with patient confidentiality, and offer clinical value, then you would be wise to pilot them.

My own NHS team find that it can be helpful to have phone reviews of patients' progress. Callbacks from nursing colleagues are particularly popular with patients in order to discuss treatment or other issues relating to their condition. We usually follow up the phone contact with a letter, which is then sent to the patient and primary care physician and added to their notes. These types of approaches may make appropriate advice more easily available for patients and reduce the need for them to attend actual appointments in the clinic. It is worth noting that at present support from the primary care commissioners and private health insurance do not cover these types of consultation. Therefore, the costs have to be covered by departmental budgets.

2 Monitor waiting times

When patients actually attend the clinic, the waiting times need to be monitored by the whole team. Staff at reception or the front desk may wish to monitor and track them over time to help identify issues and patterns. Each clinician should consider whether the running of their clinic can be improved or another type of follow-up appointment could be made use of. They can also audit follow-up appointments.

3 Aim for more shared care

Of course, alternatives have to be available and properly reimbursable. More of this type of clinical activity will happen in the future and will complement the targets of more care being shared between primary and secondary healthcare providers, more care in partnership with patients, and more care within primary care settings. For example, for blood monitoring of rheumatology patients, the blood tests are taken in primary care settings. The results are tracked in the hospital and any issues are identified. Primary and secondary care teams then liaise to make changes in treatment.

Using this type of arrangement, we have been able to reduce the total number of appointments and consultations without negatively impacting on clinical care. Of course one should never make changes that might adversely affect the health of the patients. It is a challenge to balance these concerns and goals, but it can be done.

In terms of reducing clinic demands, in our setting there are systems in primary care that screen hospital referrals. These types of screening processes filter out referrals that are not really necessary or should be seen elsewhere. For example, some orthopaedic referrals may actually need to be referred to physiotherapy or rheumatology before seeing the orthopaedic surgeon, while the main focus in the orthopaedics department is to see end stage cases to operate on.

4 Improve communication

In our experience, use of systemic patient feedback and team self-review procedures leads to more effective running of the clinics and shorter waiting times. One change we made, as a result of feedback, was to shorten the time it took to get the results of investigations to primary care physicians. The team reviewed the process and found that we could request that a copy of the results be sent to the GPs at the same time as they are sent to the clinicians. This means that patients are able to access some results via the GP's surgery and therefore need fewer clinician appointments to get their results.

Sometimes a gap in communication is caused by a problem between clinicians and patients, and it may lead to confusion that actually prolongs the course of treatment or triggers more drop-in appointments at a healthcare facility. We have addressed this problem by always copying in patients on any contact clinic visits or phone conversations.

Therefore, temporary problems related to the time taken up by patient feedback systems should eventually be balanced out by better use of clinical resources and potentially more successful courses of treatment. Furthermore, patients will gain more confidence in self-management, with the supervision of the clinical team, and a more functional healthcare system – one that puts the needs of patients first.

Patient input tools

Your patients can help you develop patient satisfaction measurement tools; you can make use of their insights and their preferences on how they wish to give feedback and the type of issues they want you to evaluate. Identifying and addressing such issues continually will assist your healthcare facility in improving and serving patients' needs better. This patient-led process can be realised using the following tools.

Preliminary questionnaires

Asking patients how they prefer to receive services, communicate with staff and discuss their issues with clinicians will give you some valuable information. Such data may be acquired through a preliminary questionnaire given to a patient before their first appointment at a healthcare facility This type of questionnaire can be completed at the same time as patients provide their general information (name, healthcare number, birthdate, address and primary care physician).

You can refine and improve your existing preliminary questionnaire by adding some questions that will determine how your patients want to experience healthcare at your facility. By recognising patterns and implementing changes that reflect the needs and wishes of your patients, you can streamline the delivery of care from the very first interaction. For example, when my NHS team identified an issue with the time it was taking to get clinic visit letters to GPs and patients, we asked patients to anonymously rate the time it took to receive the clinic letter. This enabled us to track our performance over time. In our case, it used to take *six months* and it is now down to about two weeks. We still need to improve further. Once you get into the habit of asking for feedback, it is very easy to administer a preliminary questionnaire and it takes little time for patients to complete them.

Patient feedback panels

If you have certain patients who are particularly involved with your healthcare facility (for example, because they are undergoing long-term treatments) they may be ideal candidates to be members of a small panel that meets to discuss potential improvements to healthcare delivery at your facility or institution. A clinician can lead such a panel, but it is better if it meets independently and then liaises with the healthcare facility (committee) afterwards. However it is structured, the information compiled by such a panel can be very helpful when planning changes designed to bring patients and clinicians closer together. Since panel membership will be on a voluntary basis, those who participate should be rewarded for their efforts, perhaps with refreshments at their meetings (which could be held in a spare room at your facility). If possible, their travel costs should be covered, and they should receive thank you cards, or some other polite acknowledgment of the help they have given the facility. A letter or certificate might also be issued to volunteers who assist the facility in coming up with effective ways to make healthcare interactions and service delivery more patient-led and successful. Often, a simple personal acknowledgement that individuals (patients or staff) have taken time and trouble to identify and help resolve an issue is all that is required. This is sometimes valued more than any other form of recognition.

Patient feedback surveys

Patient feedback is often measured through surveys because surveys are an excellent way to gather information that can be easily uploaded to a computer program designed to analyse such data. Surveys should ideally be straightforward and to the point. They are meant to measure a patient's satisfaction with all aspects of healthcare service delivery, from receptionists to clinicians and nurses. The main emphasis is usually placed on measuring the quality of the patient's interaction with the clinician because the quality of this interaction will determine the likelihood of the patient taking their treatment correctly and ultimately, if possible, resolving their symptoms.

Usually, a survey will ask the patient to grade certain aspects of the service using a scale of measurement, such as 1 to 5 (with one being quite dissatisfied, and five being very satisfied). Letter grades, such as A (excellent) to F (terrible) may also be used to indicate the level of satisfaction with a service. It's also possible to make things even simpler by asking patients to choose between Poor, Fair, Good or Excellent. Whatever scale of measurement you use, it's important to consider how you are going to 'crunch the numbers' or analyse your data. In most cases, a numerical scale of measurement will work best with spreadsheet programs, such as Excel, which allow users to build in formulae and create statistics.

Taking a fresh look at things and choosing to *involve* patients, rather than simply *engage* with them, can be the key to unlocking better patient experience. Only patients *really* know exactly what they want and need at every stage in the cycle of patient care, from the first greeting or phone call to the final follow-up.

Use the intelligence and emotions of your patients to design patient feedback systems that are tailor-made for them.

Mastering the fundamentals

The first step in improving patient feedback (and using that feedback to deliver better healthcare to your patients) is to understand the nature of the overall goal. Once you have decided to foster better patient feedback and patient–clinician interactions (in order to boost the potential for patient self-care and patient-led treatments), it becomes simpler to break down the task into steps. Start by formulating your mission statement or purpose, then choose your scales of measurement, types of measurement and methods of improving patient–clinician interaction.

This type of initiative is a work project, and it must be treated as such. In order to stay on schedule, you need to set up a project timeline using a computer software program such as Microsoft Project, or just handwritten notes or memos. The project timeline should include:

- A mission statement
- A chain of command
- A detailed budget
- A list of necessary supplies
- A list of involved staff and patient focus groups
- Tasks/roll-out dates
- A schedule of related special events (conferences, workshops, etc.)
- Uploading/reporting/analysis schedules for patient feedback information.

Organising the project, setting rules, training staff and sharing information will all be crucial to the success of the entire initiative.

As you can see, this is no small undertaking, but it is vital. Without effective patient feedback, the lack of communication that currently plagues patient–clinician relationships will continue to negatively affect healthcare service delivery and patient satisfaction.

At present, lack of communication is the main reason why patients feel unheard, unvalued and dissatisfied. By following the steps in this book, it will be possible to break these patterns and move into a brighter future. A change in attitude is necessary as the project rolls out – clinicians must avoid indulging in the 'ivory tower' thinking that keeps them disconnected from the thoughts and feelings of patients.

Some clinicians may feel uncomfortable with a more personal approach, as they have been trained to be emotionally detached in order to cope with the rigours of the job. After all, dealing with death, pain and chronic suffering can be quite gruelling and draining. However, developing more closeness between patient and clinician, through a more humane attitude, is really very important. Clinicians must therefore carry out some reflection and self-examination to master the fundamentals of better communication with their patients.

A change in the zeitgeist is upon us, and we must, as clinicians, step up to the challenge of the times. It is our job to provide a more personal type of care that takes into account the patient's own feelings and choices.

This holistic (or 'whole person') approach to healthcare requires us to find a balance between the traditional skills of diagnosis and treatment, and the desire to empower patients by listening to them throughout the process of healthcare delivery.

Fortunately, many clinicians have realised that they need to change their interaction methods and collect more detailed feedback. The desire to serve and help patients is always there, and this desire is helping to change the face of modern healthcare service delivery, *one appointment or treatment at a time*. Better patient feedback and more satisfactory patient–clinician interactions are vital not only to the future of the NHS but to any national health system.

Chapter 2

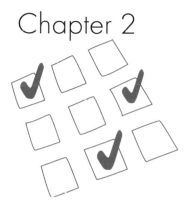

A Blueprint for Substantial Change

Providing long-term continuous patient feedback in real time is obviously challenging but it's not a pipe dream, and putting this concept into practice will undoubtedly have a positive impact on clinical practice. All our contributors agree that revisions to the healthcare system are going to accelerate, with healthcare delivery becoming increasingly focused on the needs of the patient. Better processes, responses and feedback-gathering methods lie at the heart of this 'patient involvement concept'. Over time, these adjustments will result in substantial change that alters the face of modern healthcare service delivery.

It is easiest to measure this type of substantial change in patients with long-term conditions. In the UK, long-term conditions affect about 15 million patients and account for about 80 per cent of the National Health Service's annual budget.[1] Because long-term patients use healthcare services on an ongoing basis, they provide clinicians with an effective, practical means of tracking the success and efficiency of enhanced patient feedback initiatives.

Clearly, this segment of the patient population should be studied in depth, with a focus on offering more patient-led care and better patient feedback. In fact, improving care and the quality of interactions in these vital areas should ultimately reduce the cost of treatments, while also giving patients a more satisfying, successful patient care experience. Research has shown that as many as 50 per cent of long-term care patients do not take the treatments that clinicians recommend for them.[2] In order to effect substantial change, we must grasp the underlying reasons why current feedback and interactions between patients and clinicians are failing.

[1] www.dh.gov.uk/health/category/policy-areas/nhs/long-term-conditions/

[2] World Health Organization. 2003. *Adherence to long-term therapies: evidence for action*. Geneva, Switzerland: WHO.

Why do half of patients opt out of their treatments?

There are many reasons for this, but the central fact is that somehow these patients are not persuaded to make use of the care recommended by their clinicians. In some cases, poor communication or weak rapport with healthcare service deliverers may leave patients bewildered, confused or dissatisfied, and they may let planned treatments fall by the wayside as a result. Since poor patient adherence to treatment is, in a way, an indictment of the current healthcare delivery system, it's important to consider new ways of improving the interactions between doctor and patient – as well as the entire feedback process.

Better feedback = better communication and better service

The reasons for poor patient compliance with treatments are myriad. However, as we have seen, it all tends to begin with poor or improper communication. Here are some detailed reasons why patients don't complete courses of treatment that they really need:

- Clinicians and health professionals are unable to persuade certain patients to make use of appropriate treatments for their condition.
- Poor communication leads to lack of information; patients feel that doctors do not understand, or don't care to discuss, their issues and concerns.
- Patients feel powerless during the decision-making process relating to their own health issues and conditions. They also resent being told what to do.

This limited effectiveness of care for long-term conditions would be less concerning if it did not have such dire consequences. For example, some patients who forego their treatments go on to suffer from preventable complications of their conditions, such as strokes, heart attacks, fracture of osteoporotic bones, and even death.

It is of course very important to limit the side effects of any treatment. However, in many cases some side effects will always occur. Without proper information about possible side effects and how to deal with them, patients' perception of the potential risks of taking a course of treatment will be distorted. Risks will seem amplified, and patients may imagine all manner of frightening worst-case scenarios. In such cases, better communication can reduce their fears and give them a much more accurate, realistic idea of the relative risks and benefits of their treatment.

Justified fears?

The media can provide a way for clinicians and hospitals to reach out to patients in the community. After all, many of these patients may feel some trepidation when faced with having to seek out the healthcare they need, due to fear of anaesthesia, surgery or other courses of treatment. For these patients, the idea of healthcare is fraught with peril. In fact, the healthcare system may be associated with serious fears or outright phobias, some of them justified...

The British NHS delivers approximately one million consultations per day; and around three million people are treated in the NHS every week.[3] Among this dizzying array of consultations, there is incredible variation and complexity regarding conditions and their treatments. In addition, an average of 10 per cent of inpatients in an NHS hospital will undergo an untoward event.[4] One example of a minor event would be an improper or incorrect dose of medication, or a missed dose. Another minor problem that might colour a patient's view of the healthcare delivery system and its staff would be an unforeseen delay in treatment. But at least this type of minor event, while unfortunate, will not have lasting clinical consequences.

However, not all problems related to treatment are minor. In fact, 1 in 300 inpatients suffer serious untoward events, such as having the wrong leg amputated, undergoing the wrong operation, or dying because of some other grave medical error or misunderstanding. These serious healthcare problems deter patients from seeking out the long-term care they need. These issues may also affect the way patients relate to clinicians and other healthcare staff. Fear may burden patients, preventing them from seeking out appropriate care, and who is to say that these patients don't have legitimate concerns, in the light of the statistics quoted here?

Therefore, in order to soothe their fears and re-establish rapport between patients and clinicians, the patient feedback system must be repaired. There is a need for detailed analysis to identify issues and improve communication between patients and clinicians. By taking these steps, it will be possible to improve compliance, which should lead to more positive clinical outcomes.

Small changes = significant impact

A small change, implemented over the long term, may have a very significant impact. For example, the NHS is a massive organisation of 1.3 million employees, making up a diverse group with varying skill sets and levels/types of training. With such a large enterprise, any small change that doctors and healthcare professionals put in place to improve health professional–patient interaction (even by 0.25 of 1 per cent) may make a significant difference when multiplied over the total activity of the NHS. In this way,

[3] www.nhs.uk/NHSEngland/thenhs/about/Pages/overview.aspx
[4] Vincent, C., Neale, G. & Woloshynowych, M. 2001. Adverse events in British hospitals: preliminary retrospective record review. *British Medical Journal.* **322**: 517.

small changes may result in substantial change that will probably make a real difference to important aspects of healthcare, including staff development, patient compliance, morbidity and mortality.

The patient feedback blueprint

The feedback approach is, in my opinion (and the opinion of my esteemed colleagues), the best way to standardise substantial change. We have a long-standing interest in clinical team performance and effectiveness, using strategies to reduce variations between individuals and teams to the minimum. Consistency is always our watchword as we move forward.

In 2005, we rolled out a pilot program designed to test the new concept of enhanced patient–clinician interactions and patient feedback. We have tested a variety of patient feedback questionnaires over the years. The first of these questionnaires was based on Picker Institute surveys. However, the Picker Institute documents were found to be excessively detailed. As a result, very few patients completed the questionnaires.

After this, simplicity became the priority and subsequent questionnaires were limited to just two questions. However, these surveys lacked the necessary detail and did not solicit enough information.

Clearly, a happy medium was required. A third version was therefore designed and this version was still in use in 2012. This questionnaire was one page long (see p. 21) and showed more of a *clinical* bias. The questions focus on the level of satisfaction patients experience in a variety of areas, such as waiting times, communication, the comfort of the waiting room, and so on.

The questionnaire is downloadable from the NHS Institute website.

Pre-consultation questionnaire

- www.institute.nhs.uk/images/documents/Share%20and%20network/PEN/Questionnaire%201.pdf
- www.institute.nhs.uk/images/documents/Share%20and%20network/PEN/Questionnaire%202.pdf

De-briefing tool (see p. 21)

- http://www.institute.nhs.uk/images/documents/Share%20and%20network/PEN/Questionnaire%201.pdf

The main focus of the third version of our patient feedback questionnaire was on the quality of the patient–clinician interaction. Through more effective interactions, in-clinic sessions between the patient and healthcare provider should improve the entire patient care experience. Another major benefit of better feedback and interactions is the possibility of more shared decision-making and, ultimately, improved patient outcomes.

General information

Your Age	Male	Female

Staff: Please **circle** which member of staff you saw: **Nurse Doctor Physio Other**

Place: Outpatients Inpatients General Practice Other **Date:**

	Yes	No
If still appropriate, are you taking the treatment recommended at the last clinic visit		
Would you recommend the service you received today to your friends and family? Please score out of 10, with 1 not at all to 10 highly likely		

Thank you for your help in further improving the service

What can we do better:

_____

What would have made your visit AN EXCEPTIONAL EXPERIENCE?

_____

The wait time to your next appointment is: **Satisfactory** **Too Long**

Optional: Please rate the following statements - please tick appropriate box:

	Poor	Fair	Good	Excellent	N/A
Information about the appointment was					
The manner in which I was treated by reception staff was					
The manner in which I was treated by Nurse was					
The comfort level of the waiting room was					
Length of waiting time before being seen was					
The Clinician's introduction and initial greeting was					
The opportunity I was given to express my concerns was					
The ability of the clinician to listen to me was					
The clinician's treatment and explanation of things to me was					
The respect given to my privacy was					
The time it took to receive the last clinic letter was					

Sample Questionnaire

To get started, clinicians will need to implement a briefing and de-briefing process that is not overly long-winded or complicated. Knowing how to structure the feedback process is very important, as it can have a significant impact on the success of the enterprise. In general, a short briefing before each appointment is an important aspect of 'getting the ball rolling'.

Pre-consultation sets the tone for a great interaction

At the start of each clinic, a two-minute briefing takes place, which sets out the expectations for the clinic/ward round and any exceptions. For example, in an outpatient setting, we would give a pre-consultation questionnaire to patients; and they would complete the form before visiting the clinician. This pre-consultation form enables the patient to detail exactly which symptoms are bothering them. It should also explain what a patient can expect from the consultation: a diagnosis or possible diagnosis, discussion of the prognosis, a plan for further investigation and a treatment plan.

Post-consultation provides welcome feedback

The post-consultation questionnaire should be given to patients at the end of the consultation. The attending physician, or a nurse or reception desk worker will usually hand out this questionnaire.

Using this form, patients are asked to give feedback regarding their experience in the clinic on that date; they will also be prompted to list anything that might be done better for a future appointment.

This questionnaire is anonymous, and it can be completed within a minute. The speed and anonymity of the post-consultation form should put patients at ease and streamline the patient feedback process. The completed form may be left at the reception desk in a box labelled for that purpose.

As a patient stands at the desk to make their next appointment, they can drop the feedback form in the box at the same time. This makes it quite easy and intuitive for patients to participate in the feedback process. At the end of the clinic, using the debriefing steps shown in the checklist below, the team then reviews the completed questionnaires.

Two-minute Clinical Checklist: Mahmud, T., Crump, B. 2010
Briefing at start of each clinical activity, team meet (team consists of doctor(s), nurse(s), receptionist, secretary, any observers, etc.)

1. Introduction of new member(s)

2. Any issues (waiting area, reception, other staff, offer waiting times, reading material, and drinks)

3. State the purpose of the clinic/ward round; aspiration to provide exceptional care

4. Check equipment (Notes/Investigations)

5. Patient given Pre-Consultation Questionnaire when they register at reception

6. Patients seen by the clinician and examined almost always with chaperone

7. Summarise to patient the plan regarding
   - **Investigations**
   - **Diagnosis**
   - **Treatment**
   - **Prognosis**; include relevant details in the letter (all communication copied to patients)

8. Patient invited to ask questions at end of consultation (mention Helpline, GP, written information and letter)

9. Questionnaire given to patients to complete and return to reception as they make next appointment

10. As the patient leaves the clinic room
    a. Nurse to give written information
    b. Contact details of the Helpline
    c. Remind that the letter will follow (specify ?1 week)
    d. (Deal with any issues – e.g. mis/lack of understanding/questions)

Debrief at the end of the clinic (and review feedback forms)

What went well and what could be even better

ACTIONs taken/CHANGEs made (if possible before the next clinic/ward round)

Capture thoughts/reflections worth sharing more widely

---

www.institute.nhs.uk/images/documents/Share%20and%20network/PEN/
Clinical%20Check%20list%202010%203.pdf

Debriefing tips

During debriefing, issues or improvements should be identified. Teams must reflect on their own healthcare delivery performances, and then appropriately identify any possible changes or improvements. The issues identified should be addressed as soon as possible. It's important to remember that patient feedback is optional, not mandatory. However, almost every patient will be willing to participate if the process isn't too daunting or drawn-out. Efficiency and an organised structure will assist clinicians in getting the data they want from most patients.

Each patient in a clinic will be invited to provide feedback; some 80 to 90 per cent will actually complete the questionnaire(s). The healthcare service delivery team should then begin to look at received feedback during their debriefing session. This approach provides an opportunity to gain real insight into patient experience and to recognise areas that are in need of improvement.

Sample feedback case study

Let's assume that there was feedback from a hard-of-hearing man, and he was not happy with the way health issues or treatment options were explained during his consultation. As the patient is unable to lip-read effectively (lip-reading is much harder than it looks, and many experienced lip-readers will only understand a few words in a typical sentence), other strategies could be devised to solve this communication problem during the next appointment.

For example, making sure that the patient and clinician are sitting in a well-lit area that doesn't have too much 'white noise' or 'traffic' can help a great deal. Better, more consistent eye contact and a more sensitive approach to communicating with the hard-of-hearing person can work wonders. Taking the time to jot down some notes on a pad and sharing them with the patient, while trying to speak slowly and maintain eye contact, can also make a big difference. Since many elderly patients have some degree of hearing loss (although hearing loss is actually prevalent among all generations), it's important to test out alternative ways of interacting with a hard-of-hearing patient.

Another strategy for patients who can type is for them to use a laptop or desktop computer to type questions to the doctor, who will respond in kind. For many patients who are worn out by struggling with hearing loss on a daily basis, being able to enjoy the clear understanding that comes from seeing words on a screen is a big relief. This really contributes to better communication and a more fulfilling patient–clinician interaction.

Small changes, big rewards

This new patient feedback cycle approach acknowledges the fact that small details have a great impact on the quality of interaction between healthcare professionals and patients. In almost every instance, service to patients can be improved through clearer explanations, more creative thinking and greater compassion.

Most health professionals share a sense of urgency and a wish to understand and learn from the patient's perspective by taking action *as quickly as possible*. For example, at our clinic a patient was recently observed making notes during the consultation. Before the next patient was seen, paper and pens had already been placed near seats so that other patients could take notes if they were so inclined.

This simple, commonsense approach tailors the consultation and feedback experience to the needs of patients. It clearly makes sense to implement small changes right away, and it gets results.

Bigger challenges – an example

Of course, some changes do take longer. For example, a patient once remarked that it had taken quite some time to be seen at the appropriate clinic. During a further review of similar cases, it appeared that GPs did not have a clear local pathway related to management and/or referral for patients diagnosed with Giant Cell Arteritis (GCA).

This observation led to an 18-month round of discussions and meetings between colleagues in different departments within the trust, including staff from neighbouring trusts, local primary care trusts (PCTs) and primary care branches. This group laboured to produce an efficient, PCT-wide local pathway for the initial management of GCA in each of the three population areas in the region.

PCT wide GCA pathway

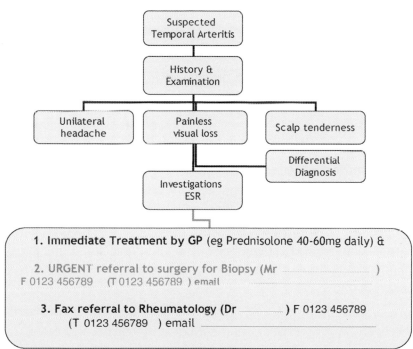

From presentation at NHS Institute website:

http://www.institute.nhs.uk/images/documents/Share%20and%20network/PEN
Long-term%20continuous%20real-time%20feedback%20-%20Taher%2Mahmud.pdf

Myriad adjustments spur substantial change

Overall, we have made more than 100 changes since the advent of our blueprint for substantial change; these were primarily basic adjustments to our offices, such as the repositioning of a weighing machine, how the door is closed during consultations, and changes to reception area seating (to provide more privacy for the registering patient).

Thanks to the blueprint for substantial change (including our feedback forms and improved patient–clinician interactions), we have better information regarding waiting times. For example, one good suggestion from a patient was the idea of placing a waiting time display board at one of the clinics. Shared decision-making with patients is also better than ever, and patients and healthcare staff are experiencing stronger rapport as a result.

Our decision-making process gives patients the power to choose their own courses of treatment, with the clinical team acting as their advisers. The blueprint for substantial change is a multi-stage process: the treatment recommendation is finalised according to the following pattern or schedule of advice, feedback and discussion:

- Pre-consultation questionnaire/appointment with the patient/post-consultation feedback
- The patient is given written information about their health issue/treatment options
- A copy of the GP's letter (summarising the in-clinic discussion) is sent to the patient
- Patient invited to call the free helpline with any questions
- Patient asked to discuss the treatment options with their GP when appropriate
- If necessary, patient may contact the consultant's office with questions, or issues may be discussed in more detail at the next clinic appointment.

The clinical treatment recommendations will probably be very clear. However, the decision to proceed with a suggested course of treatment will always rest with the patient.

Empowerment of patients lies at the heart of the blueprint for substantial change. By giving power to patients who may have formerly felt powerless when faced with the suggestions of doctors, the balance of power can be shifted and equalised. Clinicians and patients then work together for the greater good, and communication is encouraged and strengthened.

With clinicians taking on this interactive role, patients feel more valued. Furthermore, their suggestions are followed (in most cases), their concerns are heard and acted upon, and their ideas about their own treatment are taken into account. This new sense of equality between patient and clinician is a practical response to the problems that currently plague the NHS and other large-scale healthcare delivery systems.

Alert patients to all changes

To further involve our patients in the process, we strive to publish the results of our interactions and feedback on the intranet and extranet – sometimes we also post anonymous comments in the waiting area – though of course much more can still be done in this regard. However, where possible, we try to at least ensure that improvements are evident to patients. For example, changes to the layout of a waiting room will be instantly noticeable, and patients who have requested these changes will feel valued when they see their suggestions being put into practice.

Mastering the blueprint for substantial change

Most of the time and effort required to organise these changes will be in the planning phase and initial roll-out phase. In general, actually implementing the blueprint will be quite easy and intuitive. The biggest challenge is simply to adjust to a new paradigm of patient care and interaction. Instead of telling a patient what to do, a clinician must get used to considering the patient's wants and needs.

Paradigm shifts can lead to new realities. In order to address the issues that plague the modern healthcare system, clinicians, nurses and reception staff must work together in small teams, striving for a new pinnacle of healthcare service delivery.

Luckily, the blueprint demonstrated here makes it easy to get started; our team has already tested and approved these template forms and other suggestions. Of course, each department or facility may tweak the approach according to its own specifications and needs. In general, adopting the feedback process before and after consultations is the key to success in this new endeavour.

Since pre-consultations are so brief, with durations of two minutes or less, they don't represent a huge loss of time for clinicians (who are often extremely busy people). Pre-consultations are simply a new method of gauging the wishes of the patient, versus what it is actually possible to deliver during a routine appointment (in-clinic session). The post-consultation exists to reconcile the desires of the patient against what actually transpired with the clinician.

These short 'pre' and 'post' periods can offer a great deal of valuable information, and much of this information may be used to make quick changes that boost the overall satisfaction level for visitors to the healthcare facility.

More sensitivity and communication during the in-clinic appointment also reaps great dividends. Patients who once felt confused, unheard or rushed during their interactions with physicians may slowly re-orient (and improve) their opinions of general physicians and their staff.

Fears about seeking out appropriate treatments may also be eased by achieving better rapport. Barriers to communication, such as hearing loss or visual impairments, may be addressed through more creative communication methods. Patients will appreciate this humane, compassionate approach, and they will be more inclined to seek out the right treatments, based on the recommendations of their doctors.

Patient care is a science. However, it is also an art, and a relationship unlike any other. To grasp the connection between communication, interaction, feedback and better patient outcomes, doctors must see the blueprint as a whole. Each piece of the puzzle is crucial to the whole picture, and putting all the pieces together can be easier than you might imagine.

Chapter 3

The Role of Governing Organisations

Patient feedback is encouraged by governing bodies such as the General Medical Council (GMC), which monitors and registers doctors in the United Kingdom. In order to maintain a feedback system that offers benefits to long-term patients, it's important to understand the background and role of this governing organisation.

Una Lane, Director of Continued Practice and Revalidation at the General Medical Council, wrote this chapter and the perspective of a medical regulator was provided by Paul Buckley (while Director of Education and Revalidation).

Changes to patient care may be subject to scrutiny by the GMC, or (in other countries) a similar governing organisation. However, the GMC has changed a lot over the last few decades. It is now quite supportive of new techniques for bringing patients and clinicians closer together (with the aim of providing more comprehensive medical care).

It is obviously important to ensure that any new patient feedback and interaction guidelines you may introduce are aligned with the rules and regulations of the GMC. All the initiatives outlined in this book are currently aligned with the GMC's principles. While governing organisations like the GMC are usually involved with larger issues (such as resolving problems related to who should legally be allowed to practise medicine), a governing body's attitude towards changes to existing patient care guidelines will always affect the success or failure of a new initiative.

When attempting to implement changes to NHS patient feedback guidelines, a good and detailed understanding of the GMC and its role in supporting changes to healthcare service delivery and patient feedback is highly recommended.

About the General Medical Council

Here is some useful background information on this important governing body.

The General Medical Council (more commonly known as the GMC) was established in England in 1858, for the charitable purpose of 'the protection, promotion and maintenance of the health and safety of the community by ensuring proper standards in the practice of medicine'.

It is the body that is responsible for registering doctors to practise medicine in the United Kingdom. The law has granted four main functions to the GMC, under the provisions of the Medical Act (1983):

1. Keeping up-to-date registers of qualified doctors
2. Fostering good medical practice
3. Promoting high standards of medical education
4. Dealing firmly and fairly with doctors whose fitness to practise is in doubt

The GMC has four main groups of stakeholders that it works with in developing and implementing medical regulation throughout the UK. These groups are:

1. Patients and the public
2. Doctors
3. NHS and other healthcare providers
4. Medical Schools and Medical Royal Colleges

The past 25 years have been challenging for the GMC, as it has sought to find ways of improving its governance in order to facilitate the growing desire of patients (and the public) to have a greater say in who administers their medical care, what care is administered, and how such care is administered.

Throughout this period, the role and function of the GMC has evolved, as the organisation has begun to engage more with patients and the public, while also opening better channels of communication with the medical profession.

With strong support from colleagues in the four UK Departments of Health, the medical profession and the wider global community, the General Medical Council has modernised itself in a number of interesting and practical ways, as discussed below.

Good medical practice

People most commonly associate the GMC with the disciplining of doctors when there have been serious concerns about their ability to practise medicine. However, the GMC is gradually repositioning its image and purpose. The 'new' GMC is more concerned with issues relating to standards and education.

For example, the GMC has developed a guidance manual called *Good Medical Practice*, which outlines the professional standards that all doctors are expected to meet when delivering care to patients. This manual has been recognised as the leading guidance on medical practice throughout the world, and many countries have followed its example by developing similar guidance for their doctors.

The central theme of *Good Medical Practice* is the need for a proper partnership between the doctor and the patient. The old paradigm – of the doctor as the expert and the patient passively receiving the clinician's wisdom – is changing. A growing number of patients are becoming more educated about their health, through the Internet and other channels, and they are expecting to be more involved in the management of their medical care.

The standards set out in *Good Medical Practice* emphasise the importance of doctors working *with* patients. This manual clearly outlines what the GMC expects from the doctor/patient relationship.

GMC governance: Adding lay members to the Council

The theme of change is also reflected in recent amendments to the governance structures of the GMC. In the past, the GMC predominantly supported the idea of professional self-regulation, which meant that most of the GMC Council members were registered medical doctors.

In 2009, the GMC proposed a move away from a self-regulatory business model and towards a more balanced model, with equal numbers of lay representatives and medical representatives. This reorganisation proved to be challenging for many doctors, who found it difficult to accept that they would have less influence over the regulation of their profession, and that they would have to share this role with lay members who were not medically qualified.

However, the GMC has been established for some time now, and it is clearly showing that a partnership between patients, the public and the medical profession can provide effective governance of healthcare regulation for the future.

Patient reference community

In addition to the 12 lay representatives sitting on the GMC, the Council has taken steps to engage more widely with patients and the public regarding its policies and plans for the future. In 2011, a patient reference community was established, with 25 patient and public members. These people are regularly asked to consider (or review) new GMC policy ideas, and to give feedback from a patient's perspective about how these policies could be improved or might work in practice.

The GMC uses this community as a sounding board at an early stage, to get a sense of whether a proposed policy is sensible, equitable and generally going in the right direction. Although it is early days for this patient reference community, it seems to be an invaluable resource for the GMC as they strive to develop plans for improving local clinical governance (and doctors' annual appraisal) through a new regulatory mechanism called revalidation.

Revalidation

Revalidation is a new type of medical regulation that will require all doctors to demonstrate (on a regular basis) that their knowledge is up to date and they are fit to practise. Historically, once a doctor was registered with the GMC, they would be able to practise medicine without any regular checks, unless something serious happened and they were reported to a regulatory authority for disciplinary action.

However, a number of high-profile cases in the 1980s and 1990s revealed that a range of problems involving doctors and other healthcare professionals had not been reported to the relevant authorities, or had not been dealt with as they should have been. These cases prompted a change in the way the GMC approached registration. It is no longer enough for a doctor to say, 'Trust me – I am a doctor on the register'. Instead, clinicians need to demonstrate, through an ongoing process called revalidation, that they are keeping their skills and knowledge up to date, and that they are fit to practise medicine in the UK.

Revalidation will require doctors to collect patient feedback about their practice through surveys. Patients will have the opportunity to provide feedback on the performance of their doctors, and this information will be discussed at the doctor's annual appraisal. It will also be considered during the revalidation process. Since 2011, systematic revalidation has been gradually put in place. Now that this process is complete, patients will be able to look at the medical register and other professional registers to check a doctor's qualifications, as well as their revalidation status.

Patient safety is the number one priority

Patient safety is a cornerstone of GMC business, and patients (and the general public) are one of the four main stakeholder groups linked to the GMC's work. Over the last few decades, the GMC has ensured that it has more lay and patient input in its governance and policy development. It has also developed guidance and new regulatory processes that prioritise the needs of patients in their relationships with doctors.

Finally, the GMC is developing systems to encourage patients to give feedback on the medical care that they receive, so that their opinions and suggestions can influence and direct improvements in the quality of care delivered to patients now and in the future.

Committed to 'good medical practice', the General Medical Council has worked to educate the public about exactly what role patients can play in ensuring that they receive the best possible healthcare. In fact, the GMC's promotional materials include a list of promises from doctors to patients. This honourable 'agreement' is a good way of showing that doctors are now (more than ever) committed to giving patients the very best communication, respect and treatment.

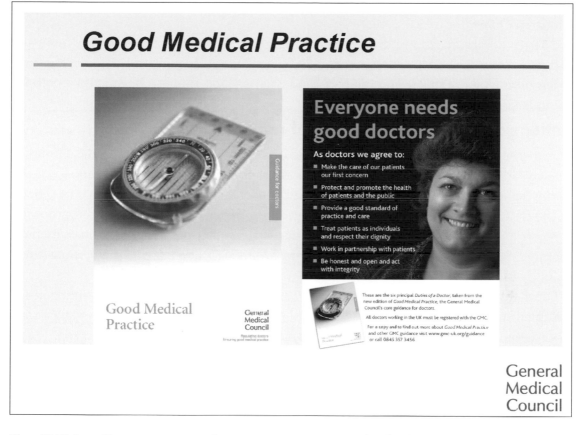

The GMC is still most commonly seen as a governing body that 'polices' doctors who have 'gone wrong' in some way. However, as the above poster shows, the GMC's role is changing and broadening.

It is true that a large part of the GMC budget is still spent on 'fitness to practise' (i.e. questions that may arise regarding whether or not some doctors should still be registered). But during the next few years, the GMC expects to see much more public focus on the education standards work that they are undertaking.

A new partnership

The central theme of the GMC's revamped mission statement is clearly the need for a proper partnership between doctor and patient. The old paradigm of the patient being a passive recipient, and the doctor possessing all medical knowledge, is now being swept away by technological change, which has made information much more widely available. However, the Internet is a flawed medical educator, as many of its information sources are sketchy at best. People may learn more about health issues and problems and see themselves as lay experts, but the information sources they find on the Internet will vary enormously in terms of reliability and this will affect whether or not they are properly educated online.

Better communication between doctor and patient can cut through any confusion that may arise. The GMC features a detailed website that doctors and patients can visit to learn more about this governing body and its impact on modern healthcare – both for patients and clinicians.

Better governance – principles of redesign

This theme of change is also reflected in the governance of the General Medical Council. A few years ago, the GMC was a predominantly *medical* body, and self-regulation was the norm. Self-regulation required that a majority of doctors appeared on the governing body of the GMC and other health regulation authorities. Three years ago, the GMC proposed a move away from that design; the new goal became a 50% lay and 50% medical membership. Of course, some doctors found it difficult to accept this new, more equal 'balance of power'.

The Council is more established now and this new structure is becoming more accepted; new governance of healthcare regulation demonstrates the need for a partnership between patients, the public and the profession.

However, there still needs to be more representation by lay people on the GMC. One step the GMC has taken, as discussed earlier, is to establish a patient reference community or committee to engage with patients, the public and doctors (see p. 31). GMC representatives may ask the reference committee, for example, 'Is this the sort of thing we need to be doing, in your opinion?'

The new relationship between the patient reference committee and GMC policy development is an embryonic idea that requires further testing. Ultimately, the needs of the GMC's primary stakeholders must be aligned with both parties and their decision-making.

Revalidation is being completely redesigned in such a way that individual doctors will need to demonstrate on a regular basis that they are up to date and fit to practise. Historically, the model dictated that registration with an organisation such as the GMC meant that you were qualified up to a certain point in time. The assumption was that you would still be qualified 20 or 30 years later, unless you had been reported to a regulatory authority for some alleged offence.

This new era of multi-source feedback and governance is giving patients a voice in how (and by whom) their healthcare is delivered. However, the concept of revalidation also causes stress for doctors, who are already under significant pressure as they go about their daily duties.

Patient feedback can of course be negative as well as positive. Negative feedback can potentially harm a clinician's career, because it may trigger problems in becoming revalidated, based on the new rules. Therefore, for many doctors, the desire to participate in better feedback systems may be counteracted by anxiety about the possibility of negative feedback and its effects. Many of these clinicians may long for the simplicity of the old system.

However, the balance of power has shifted, and it is not likely to shift back. At this point, it is almost always in a doctor's best interests to listen to feedback carefully, to make changes that take patient feedback into account, and to improve the quality of patient–clinician interactions. Since the new rules are probably here to stay, the best defence against attack is to work together with patients for the greater good.

As you can see, there is a dichotomy here. Clinicians must seek out better patient feedback in order to serve patients more effectively. However, the feedback they solicit may be used against them in some way. This tension is central to the impact of governance on national healthcare systems, such as the NHS.

Other professional bodies regulate the conduct of particular health professionals (such as the Nursing and Midwifery Council, the General Dental Council, and so on), and patient feedback is becoming increasingly important for all these organisations as well.

Chapter 4

The Psychology of Better Communication

To improve communication between patients and clinicians, it is vital to gain an understanding of the psychology of communication.

The first point is that all communication requires a sender and a receiver. The way senders and receivers exchange signals may be verbal or non-verbal. Both types of cues, along with other important variables (such as the relative comfort, privacy and layout of a room), will have a significant impact on the success of any patient–clinician interaction. To assess how effectively you communicate with patients, you need to consider the way you send and receive signals during your working day.

Most healthcare professionals want to communicate well and to engage with their patients. However, certain obstacles to communication may arise, as discussed below.

Dealing with barriers to communication

Reasons for less-than-perfect interactions with patients may include stress, overscheduling, cultural differences, disability (on either side), language barriers and general differences of opinion. The first section in this chapter offers tips on how to overcome all these barriers.

Stress

Stress is easier to deal with if you take the time to analyse its root cause. For instance, if family problems are leaving you feeling tense at work (and less able to interact with patients successfully), it's important to recognise the problem and deal with it. Seeking therapy, getting more sleep or exercise, taking supplements and improving your nutrition may strengthen your body and mind, making it easier to deal with problems that interfere with patient–clinician communication.

If your feeling of stress is work-related, you need to consider ways to ease the pressure. For example, shift changes, delegation or enhancing your skills (through reading, self-reflection, or feedback from patients and your team) may all help to relieve stress at your place of employment.

Of course, a certain amount of stress is part of normal life. However, when stress gets out of control, it can lead to anxiety and depression, and make it difficult to function effectively. When you are clearly under a great deal of pressure, your patients will sense this and will feel less able to connect with you.

Overscheduling

This is a big problem in larger healthcare systems. Sometimes it may seem that there are not enough hours in the day to take care of all your patients in the way they deserve. You may feel consternation about the ticking clock and a waiting room crowded with patients. Waiting times will almost always be a factor in overscheduling woes, causing patients to become irritated and thus increasing your stress levels. Since some or all of your patients may be 'walk-ins', it's impossible to eliminate the possibility of some overscheduling.

If you are feeling overscheduled, you may be rushing through clinical sessions. You may even be (unwittingly) sending the message that you don't have time to interact sufficiently with patients or to solicit feedback from them. In some cases, clinicians may actually be afraid to ask for feedback because they fear the response!

However, there are solutions to this problem as well. With proper tracking and analysis of waiting times, patient health issues and follow-up appointments, it may be possible to streamline the flow of patients to your clinic.

Cultural differences

Sometimes cultural differences affect the way clinicians interact with their patients. Dealing with these issues requires education. Learning more about other cultures and their concepts of manners and etiquette can be very useful. Understanding gender roles in other societies may also be helpful.

Luckily, in the age of the Internet, it's quite easy to search for information about other cultures. The more you know, the easier it will be to build a rapport with people from other backgrounds. Religion, in particular, may affect the way a patient views treatment – for example, Jehovah's Witnesses don't believe in having blood transfusions; they prefer to leave cures 'in God's hands'.

The more you learn about other cultures and religions, the more you will be able to promote a spirit of diversity and multiculturalism while taking care of your patients. Documentaries, magazine articles, newspaper stories and blogs or websites about other cultures are all excellent resources. Your own knowledge will increase over time and you can always ask advice from colleagues if in doubt.

Disability

Disabilities, on the part of clinicians or patients, may affect the way patients and healthcare staff interact. Hearing loss is a primary cause of difficulties in communication, and deafness is a fairly common disability. Its impact may be quite subtle, with the patient not making clear that they have this disability and the clinician looking down, making notes and thereby making it impossible for the patient to lip-read.

Visual impairments, stuttering and mobility issues may also create barriers. Likewise, psychological problems, such as Schizoid Personality Disorder or Asperger's and other types of autism, may present significant communication challenges.

However, it is always possible to overcome these obstacles by means of creative thinking and different ways of communicating. Every type of common disability should be considered, and a list of acceptable and appropriate alternative communication methods should be implemented.

An obvious starting point is to talk to people with a disability about what works best for them. An initial conversation exploring the disabled person's favourite modes of communicating will set the tone for a good patient–clinician interaction. Sometimes the patient may have a carer, relative or friend attending to assist with communication, which can be very beneficial during the consultation. However, you should still make a point of speaking to the patient at all times so that they remain at the centre of the consultation and have an opportunity to direct their own care and treatment choices.

Taking the time to break down these barriers will help you grow as a clinician, and it may lead to the implementation of some excellent processes that change the way you communicate with disabled patients.

Language barriers

It's very hard to speak to someone who isn't fluent in your native tongue. Of course, learning other languages will alleviate this problem, but learning several languages is time-consuming and will not be feasible for most clinicians. Fortunately, there are other options.

Firstly, you should discuss with your patient the possibility of getting an interpreter. This interpreter could be a family member or friend, or someone else the patient trusts. An interpreter may even be a member of your staff who is fluent in a certain language. However, interpreters will be privy to the patient's healthcare information and other personal matters. It is therefore important that everyone understands the pros and cons before an interpreter is used.

It may also be possible to get frequently used leaflets and patient information sheets translated into other languages commonly used where your healthcare facility operates.

Differences of opinion

It is difficult to counsel someone who displays a hostile attitude or openly disagrees with your methods or diagnoses. However, differences of opinion are inevitable. The way you deal with dissent from a patient will be part of what defines you as a clinician; you must remain professional and do your very best to understand and respect the patient's perspective and explain the need for treatment in terms that will make sense to them.

Bear in mind that differences of opinion can actually be very good learning experiences – your patient may be expressing a common dislike that many other patients share. Therefore, you should carefully consider the patient's point of view and try to discuss their concerns in a caring and compassionate manner.

Taking a constructive learning approach to understanding every patient's views will help you turn a potentially negative interaction into a positive learning experience – for both you *and* the patient.

Improving communication

Getting past these barriers will allow clinicians to achieve more effective communication, which is vital in establishing good patient feedback. Once communication barriers have been addressed, healthcare professionals need to consider the way they use language, body language and other psychological cues to get their point across. They must also learn to read the non-verbal cues they receive from patients.

Reading non-verbal cues from patients

Non-verbal cues include things like flushing or blushing (cheeks and/or throat) in response to a statement or action from another person; this type of reaction is known as a *sign*. Other signs might include shaking or trembling (if this is not a symptom of an underlying health problem), or fidgeting. These signs all indicate embarrassment, nervousness or some other form of agitation or stress.

If patients are giving you signs, you must listen to their words, but also pay close attention to what they are *not* telling you, by observing their non-verbal cues. Sometimes taking the time to study a patient's signs can be very revealing.

Not every clinician will be perceptive enough to analyse underlying emotions from signs. However, doctors are trained to observe carefully in order to diagnose correctly and most are therefore likely to be excellent and intuitive judges of the signs relating to the psychology of communication. Learning to study signs is one of the hallmarks of a superior patient–clinician interaction.

Controlling your own non-verbal cues

Observing a patient's signs, while listening to their words and responding in kind, can be difficult, as you will also need to consider any signs *you* may be giving to a patient.

After all, our understanding of signs and signals may often be subconscious, and some people will naturally 'feel' the effects of another person's signs and signals. For example, if a doctor glances at their watch frequently during an appointment, this overt signal may deter a patient from explaining their health issues and related concerns. The patient may intuit that the doctor is in a hurry, or even bored by the discussion.

Therefore, the signs you send out during such an interaction can have an enormous bearing on the success of a patient feedback improvement initiative. The goal is to be totally present, in the moment, when spending time with a patient. No distractions should be allowed to enter your mind, as patients will almost certainly feel these distractions through your non-verbal cues. In this sense, your body language is the key to positive interactions that will garner helpful patient feedback. These positive interactions will in turn lead to successful courses of treatment and patient care experiences.

Using the right body language

To make the most of a patient–clinician interaction, you need to use body language that reinforces your authority and trustworthiness, while still putting the patient at ease. It's important to show a caring face, and to back up your words and tone with the right body language. Here are some tips on how to make your body language more positive.

Watch your posture

Set the tone of your interaction by exhibiting good posture – slumping or hunching of the spine sends negative signals to patients. Walk (or sit) tall, and you will exude confidence.

Shake hands properly

Shaking hands may be a good way to spread germs, but it's also a popular social greeting that carries a strong psychological message. If you shake hands with patients, make sure you use an appropriately firm grip. Your handshake should not be crushing – it should never hurt the patient. However, it should never be clammy or weak either. It should be strong enough to send a message of strength and authority. Always maintain eye contact while shaking hands – smiling helps, too.

Smile more

Smiling is a great way to put patients at ease, as people who smile always seem more approachable. Of course you don't need to grin your way through an in-clinic session that deals with someone's health problems! But you should make a point of smiling whenever it is tactful or appropriate. Think about your current in-clinic sessions – are you smiling enough?

Train yourself to smile a few times, and try to be as genuine as possible. You may find you sometimes need to 'fake it until you feel it'. However, the more you get used to using a smile as a social tool with patients, the more you will see the value of this practice. A genuine, happy smile will always help you bond with another person, and it's so easy to do.

Maintain steady eye contact

The eyes are the windows of the soul, according to the old saying. They allow you to express a plethora of emotions without saying a word. However, if you don't maintain steady eye contact, you may be under-using one of your most important communication tools.

Eye contact during consultations and other interactions sends a message of receptiveness, confidence and strength. Studies have shown that powerful members of society tend to influence others by using a great deal of eye contact while they speak.

Conversely, timid patients may 'shy away' from meeting your eyes during an appointment. This is usually due to feelings of powerlessness, which you may be able to assuage once you know about them. Of course, fears about a health issue or disease may be weighing the patient down psychologically.

Certain patients with personality disorders, such as Avoidant Personality Disorder sufferers, may live with a profound lack of self-esteem that makes eye contact painful or uncomfortable. However, even these patients will appreciate the effort you make to connect with them. In fact, they are the ones who need your authority, knowledge and warmth the most.

Always attempt to increase rapport by meeting a patient's eyes regularly; and use this close bonding to get a better sense of who the patient is, and what they need and want.

Avoid bad habits

Certain behaviours, such as jamming your hands into your pockets, will send the 'wrong message'. Other bad habits include chewing gum, fiddling with objects (such as pens or paper clips) and holding onto coffee cups or other objects while talking to patients.

Generally, holding objects (such as clipboards, pagers, phones or files) in front of you will create a psychological barrier that stops you connecting with others. Chewing gum or fidgeting will give you an air of immaturity and/or impatience. Having your hands in your pockets will send a message that you are sealed off from the patient in some way.

Another common bad habit is touching your own face while talking to others. For example, touching your chin is commonly viewed as being indicative of lying. Many people believe that those who touch their faces frequently in a conversation may not be telling the truth.

Crossing your arms in front of you will also put patients off. This type of body language bad habit may seem innocuous, but it will send a message that you are creating a safe area between you and a patient, and thus sealing yourself off from them.

Knowing how body language is interpreted by psychologists and subconsciously understood by patients can be very useful. For example, once you know which bad habits to avoid, you can also notice these bad habits in others, and spot them in the form of non-verbal cues that help you to understand your patients a little better. Of course, the psychology of communication isn't everything. It's obviously also important to have in-depth discussions of the treatment options and offer patients a chance to express their own healthcare preferences. For an optimum interaction that results in excellent feedback, you need to consider both verbal and non-verbal cues and really talk (and listen) to the patient in a meaningful way.

Deciphering the patient's verbal cues

Speech is about more than the words that are spoken; the way speech is delivered can also be quite telling. Different verbal cues, such as tone, volume and intensity, will all be very revealing. While tone is often self-explanatory (in that we can ascertain quite easily whether or not someone is angry, sad or elated, simply by hearing their tone of voice), other verbal cues may be less obvious. Here are some aspects to consider when listening to a patient.

Pressured speech

If a patient's speech seems too rapid and too loud, and you have difficulty getting a word in, there may be an underlying psychological cause, such as bipolar disorder. However, there is always the possibility that pressured speech is simply the result of anxiety or nerves.

Many patients do feel ill at ease with their clinicians. If you can, try to soothe the patient with the correct, welcoming body language and a calm, friendly tone of voice. If pressure of speech continues without decreasing at all, it may be a signal that the patient is experiencing bipolar hypomania.

Repetition

The repetition of certain words or sentences may also be a signal of an underlying psychological condition, such as autism. Repeating words over and over again is a red flag symptom of this disorder in children and adults. However, you should bear in mind that this could also be due to the patient simply being nervous or having a stammer.

Distancing language

This type of language may be something you need to watch out for yourself, as clinicians often tend to use distancing language to describe disturbing health conditions or symptoms. An example of distancing language would be saying that someone 'exsanguinated', rather than explaining that they 'died due to massive blood loss'. Obviously, distancing language does serve a purpose; it can protect others from being emotionally disturbed. However, too much use of distancing language can create a chasm between you and a patient.

Some patients may have had limited educational opportunities; using difficult, technical or distancing vocabulary may therefore overcomplicate interactions and leave them confused about what has actually been said. Plain speech is a vital tool in better patient–clinician interactions. It's very important to speak plainly, and to avoid distancing language where possible.

Patients who use distancing language themselves may be too timid or embarrassed to explain their physical symptoms plainly. They may use euphemistic distancing language in order to put a more 'respectable' face on things. If you find that a patient is retreating into distancing language, be sensitive and try to draw them out a little. The chances are that it will be a relief for them to discuss things in plainer terms. However, bear in mind that every patient is different, and their reasons for employing distancing language will vary accordingly.

In some cases the patient may be very reluctant to use plain language and should not be pressurised to do so. For example, some elderly people may find it utterly impossible to use certain terms, especially if the doctor is of the opposite sex. In such cases, it might be worth asking a female patient if she would prefer to speak to a female doctor, and a male patient if he would prefer to consult a male clinician.

Tone of voice

Often, tone of voice is quite easy for almost anyone to decipher. After all, we go through life adjusting our tone of voice to suit different people and a dizzying array of social situations. However, it's always good to consider the tone of voice you use with patients, and also to consider the patient's own tone. In general, your voice should not be too flat or monotonous; it should also not be too loud or dominating.

The 'middle of the road' is a good analogy for the correct tone of voice to use during in-clinic interactions; medium volume and medium inflection will be best. If a patient speaks too loudly, they may suffer from undiagnosed hearing loss – it's important to watch for these verbal cues and consider them. If a patient is too softly spoken, they may be shy in a clinician's presence. Modulating your own voice to speak clearly, at an acceptable volume, is very important.

Providing the right environment for communication

Now that we've examined some important aspects of the psychology of communication, we can consider the in-clinic setting and atmosphere. There are a number of environmental elements that may affect the success of a conversation between a doctor and a patient.

These include:

- **Temperature**: Is the room too cold or too hot?

- **Privacy**: Can others hear what is being said? In-clinic rooms should be private and soundproofed to reassure the patient that the conversation will be confidential. Even a door that is slightly ajar may hinder a patient's desire to confide in a physician.

- **Noise**: White noise from machines, or noise from a nearby waiting room, may annoy a patient and make it harder for them to communicate with a clinician. For the hearing-impaired, white noise is a huge problem that definitely gets in the way of positive interaction.

- **Cleanliness**: The cleanliness of the room is an important factor in patient–clinician interactions; rooms should be immaculate whenever possible. Any waste or used materials from the last patient's examination should be disposed of, or moved out of sight.

- **Comfort**: As patients may have to wait in the examination room for the doctor to arrive, magazines should be available, as well as a comfortable chair where they can relax until the clinician arrives. Bear in mind that medical appointments make some patients nervous, and if they are feeling unwell they may be quite tense or restless. Making them wait for a long period in a sterile room, with nothing to do, is a bad idea and may well affect the success of the patient–clinician interaction.

- **Odours**: Odours should be neutral. Always avoid wearing heavy scents (such as perfume, cologne, aftershave, body lotions and hand creams) when you are taking care of patients, who may have allergies or sensitivities to fragrance. The cleansers used to wash hands and tidy the exam room should also have a neutral and inoffensive scent.

Spending more time with each patient

Studies have shown that patients really respect and believe in doctors who go out of their way to provide them with all the information they need. These clinicians don't cut corners – they take things slowly, spend sufficient time with each patient, and carefully explain (in plain English) everything the patient needs to know about their health problem and treatment options.

Clearly, patients are looking for more in-depth interaction with their clinicians, and short, abrupt in-clinic sessions are likely to exacerbate distrust between doctor and patient. With waiting times getting ever longer, there can be real pressure to speed up the whole process of seeing patients and assigning courses of treatment. However, although this may appear to make things quicker in the short term, it actually contributes to the degradation of the entire healthcare system in the long run.

Sometimes patients leave healthcare facilities feeling hard done by, confused or badly informed. They wonder why the doctor didn't give them more than a few moments to voice their concerns and discuss important health matters. After all, national health systems are supposed to function for the good of the people...

In fact, resisting the pressure to speed up, and instead spending more time with each patient, may lead to more successful patient outcomes. This will benefit your practice in the long term, as patients will be more likely to experience positive interaction and good communication, leading to more effective patient care. Therefore, spending more time on each appointment may be an excellent idea – even an extra five to ten minutes per patient can make an enormous difference.

Consider adding a five-minute block of time to each in-clinic session, and be certain to allow for a two-minute pre-consultation session as well. For only seven minutes of additional time per patient, you can get a more detailed, in-depth sense of what they expect, and how you can deliver the desired results. A post-consultation feedback form can be given to the patient afterwards – and they can fill this form out while they wait at the front desk to book their next appointment.

A longer in-clinic session gives clinicians time to employ the techniques discussed in this chapter. Doctors will be able to monitor their own body language, speak clearly, and watch and listen for verbal and non-verbal cues. The extra five minutes should be specifically tailored to foster better rapport between the patient and doctor. Since revalidation is in the offing (see p. 32), it's vital that clinicians learn to refine their in-clinic sessions and their own styles of communication with patients.

Gaining an understanding of the psychology of communication can add richness and a new dimension to a typical in-clinic visit. In human interactions, there are always several layers of communication (including subtext, body language, tone of voice, intensity of speech and expressions). These will all affect the quality of the interaction and whether it is a positive or negative experience for the participants.

Understanding and thinking about these elements can add value to your practice of medicine, and may well result in positive feedback from patients, who will enjoy the extra time you spend getting to know them and serving their needs. This enhanced communication will bridge a gap that has been widening for decades, as the system has buckled under the pressure of too many patients, not enough funding, and burnt-out, stressed medical personnel.

By adding a little extra time to each appointment, and considering the psychology of communication, clinicians can bring more emotional intelligence to their interactions with patients. Practising medicine requires knowledge, skill, observation and decision-making. When physicians are busy thinking about all these different aspects, the emotional elements of the job (which are very real) sometimes tend to fall by the wayside. Patients can easily end up feeling devalued by being pushed through the system too quickly. This is why it is so vital for clinicians to slow things down, and give detailed, in-depth care to every single patient.

Better communication is really the only way to heal a system that is strained, and perhaps broken in places. A more humane approach is vital to the regeneration of the National Health Service, and other, similar national healthcare organisations.

Improving your listening skills

With all this in mind, let's explore some techniques for improving your listening skills, as listed below.

Avoiding pitfalls

The worst listeners fall into a series of traps that derail conversations. Here are some examples of these pitfalls.

Rehearsal

The next time you're in an in-clinic session with a patient, think about your own listening style. While the patient is speaking, are you focusing on them completely, or are you mentally rehearsing what you are going to say next? This type of mental rehearsal can pull your mental focus away from the other person, and it may also give you a distracted air. Rehearsing speech while someone else is speaking is definitely one of the pitfalls that surfaces in interactions. Avoiding this trap will help you become a better listener.

Self-referencing

Bringing the conversation around to yourself can be a mistake, as it makes patients think you are only concerned with yourself and your own experiences. If you have a habit of self-referencing during patient–clinician interactions, try to rephrase your words to remove any references to yourself. It's quite easy to slip into these traps, and it can colour the way patients see you. You may find it hard at first to constantly monitor spontaneous speech to get rid of such pitfalls, but it will become natural in time. Bad listening habits will be broken as you learn to take in what the other person is saying with a focused mind, and respond without self-referencing

Subconscious filters

When listening to another person, it's very easy to impose subconscious filters. This sort of filtering will affect both you and the patient, as filtering only allows the listener to tune in to certain key words or phrases. Usually, listeners filter because they are tired or simply weary of a conversation. They 'tune out' (whether consciously or subconsciously) what doesn't seem to be valuable. Of course, filtering will therefore cause you to miss many verbal and non-verbal cues, and it may affect your relationship with the patient. During in-clinic sessions, it's vital to be 'on task' and focused on every single word. After all, patients have very little time to spend with their doctors, and they need to feel valued and heard during each appointment.

Developing good listening techniques

The best listening is *active listening*. During normal interactions, most people only catch between 25 and 50 per cent of what the other person is saying. This is partly because people begin to give in to the pitfalls we discussed earlier. In order to listen actively, it's vital to open your mind, focus completely on the other person, and make a point of listening as wholeheartedly as possible.

Since doctors are usually face-to-face with patients during in-clinic sessions, they are in an ideal setting for superior active listening. This type of listening can lead to very successful patient–clinician interactions, as long as all barriers to good communication are lowered. Distractions should be eliminated, and you should utilise your knowledge of the psychology of effective communication, as discussed earlier. Here are some ways to ensure that your listening is as active as possible.

Show interest

Fidgeting or doing other things (multi-tasking) during an interaction is a bad idea, but there are certain movements that clinicians *should* make to let patients know that they are listening to them. For example, nodding or smiling (when appropriate) can provide excellent visual cues that reassure the patient.

These mannerisms will make the patient feel that their words are registering, and that their concerns and thoughts are seen as valid. Building confidence and dignity in patients is what better communication is all about. Let your patient know that you care – display your active listening through movements designed to boost the positive elements of a patient–clinician interaction.

Offer feedback

This book is all about *getting* feedback, not giving feedback. However, giving feedback is also important. During active listening, making small comments on what the person has said will spur them on and enable them to feel comfortable when expressing their feelings and ideas.

Never interrupt, as interrupting is rude. Instead, wait for a lull, chime in with some feedback about what the patient has said, and then ask them to 'go on…' and explain more about how they are feeling, or their concerns about a proposed course of treatment. Interspersing nods, smiles and feedback can be an excellent way to keep energy flowing between a patient and a doctor during a clinic appointment.

You may also want to encourage reception staff and nurses to embrace the concept of active listening as they go about their duties.

Always be polite

In a culture of rushed interactions, where impatience and even outright rudeness are not uncommon, good manners are at a premium. Most patients will appreciate any form of kindness, and good manners are a wonderful way to show compassion and a graceful, grateful attitude.

Good manners include always being politically correct. Nothing 'off-colour' or controversial should ever be discussed during the chat that may precede an in-clinic session. 'Hot-button topics' that should never be discussed include politics and religion.

Some people may think that manners are old-fashioned but they are always charming and will make people feel valued. You are not in a patient–clinician relationship to charm, but a little sweetness will go a long way towards breaking down barriers to great communication. 'Honey catches more flies than vinegar,' as the old saying goes. Of course, you must still be professional – no hint of flirtation should ever enter the proceedings. The right balance may be hard to achieve at first, but warming up your approach to patient–clinician interactions can be very helpful. In a nutshell, many patients are currently not satisfied with the quality of interaction they are receiving. In many cases, things therefore need to change to please the patient, and to get good feedback.

Being polite involves holding doors open, addressing a person correctly, saying please and thank you, and generally going out of your way to put another person at their ease. From inquiring whether the temperature of the examination room is comfortable for the patient, to asking them whether they had to travel far to the clinic, good manners will put your patients at ease and make them feel special. It's not your job to make friends with patients, but warmth and genuine concern are absolutely appropriate.

Give patients an outlet

Good listening skills will soothe patients and offer them a vital outlet. Everyone suffering from health issues is subject to stress and worry, and they may feel all alone with their concerns. In the case of the elderly, there may be a degree of isolation, as they might be widowed or somehow cut off from others due to loss of hearing, sight or mobility.

By being a good listener and a sensitive human being, you can do your job well, while also providing patients with an outlet. Your active listening will encourage 'venting', which releases pressure and gives patients a sense of release or relief.

Good therapists are trained to listen carefully and with exceptional skill – part of their job is to be an effective sounding board for their clients. Clinicians may wish to borrow the techniques of skilled therapists by using careful listening techniques that offer patients the chance to express their thoughts and emotions without fear or judgement. This aspect of excellent listening can add depth to patient–clinician interactions.

Conclusion

Good communication is a skill that many gregarious people achieve naturally. Other, more introverted personality types may struggle to exchange thoughts and ideas without nervousness or awkwardness. However, anyone, from bold Type-As to shy, retiring folk, can learn how to listen more effectively. The skills associated with the psychology of good communication can be learnt through books, online tutorials, documentaries on good listening, and many other channels. You only need the motivation to acquire these skills – and you will be able to do so.

By considering verbal and non-verbal cues, clinicians can tap into a deeper understanding of their patients, and add value to in-clinic visits. Patients will walk away feeling understood, and will have all the facts they need to make informed decisions about courses of treatment and other health-related recommendations.

In the past, many doctors may have seemed detached from patients, partly because they have focused on their symptoms or bodies alone, without giving any attention to their thoughts, feelings and emotions. Now, a more holistic approach to healthcare is required. The well-being of the patient is the top priority, and patients have strongly indicated that they want better listening and more in-depth conversations with their doctors. They want plain language, compassion and choices.

All these requirements can be fulfilled through better patient feedback. Pre-consultation sessions will give clinicians valuable information about exactly what patients want out of their appointment. Clinicians can then use this information during the in-clinic visit to ensure that patients receive what they require.

Good listening techniques and knowledge of the psychology of communication can be combined to provide patients with a more satisfying examination. After the in-clinic session, patients will be free to leave additional feedback through a quick and simple questionnaire. The healthcare team can then scan this form to see how a patient responded to their clinician, as well as other members of a team.

Instantly, doctors and other staff will have what they need to analyse an interaction, and to improve matters next time round (if necessary). The beauty of better patient feedback is that the gains are consistent and never-ending. Improvements designed to benefit a particular patient are likely to benefit many others as well. In this way, the system will be automatically adapted to meet patients' needs more effectively, and changes will be made quickly and efficiently.

Chapter 5

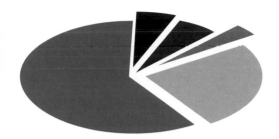

Healing the Healthcare System

In this chapter, we'll take a look at some expert advice on healing the healthcare system. The perspective of the Chief Executive in a large, acute hospital group is provided by Glenn Douglas, Maidstone and Tunbridge Wells NHS Trust.

Lately, the NHS has received some bad press, specifically relating to patient care standards that are below par, as well as outbreaks of illness that may be caused by poor cleanliness at NHS hospitals. This adverse media attention (which has escalated over the past few years) may well be one reason for the heightened awareness of the importance of patient satisfaction and patient feedback. In fact, the whole concept of the General Medical Council's revalidation process is perhaps a natural response to the current image of the NHS and its clinicians and staff.

At some point, all national healthcare systems will falter, mistakes will be made, and governing bodies will react accordingly. The Clostridium difficile outbreak that occurred between 2004 and 2006 at Maidstone and Tunbridge Wells NHS Trust (MTW) provides a worst-case scenario, from which many lessons can be learnt. These tragic events can be used to inspire new progress and better healthcare in the future. Before a healthcare system can be healed, damage must be realistically assessed.

With all this in mind, Glenn Douglas has agreed to share his insights. Glenn was appointed Chief Executive of the Maidstone and Tunbridge Wells (MTW) NHS Trust in January 2008. Before joining MTW, Glenn worked as CEO of Ashford and St Peter's Hospitals NHS Trust. He joined the MTW Trust immediately before the publication of the notorious Healthcare Commission report into the Clostridium difficile outbreak.

What is Clostridium difficile?

Clostridium difficile (C. difficile) bacteria are part of a group of bacteria that trigger tetanus and botulism. This type of C. difficile bacterium occurs in a couple of forms, one of which is an active, infectious form. Active C. difficile bacteria can only survive for a finite period in a typical environment. The second type of non-active C. difficile bacterium is in spore form, and is considered non-infectious. However, spores can be taken into the human body through ingestion. When this occurs, inactive bacteria may be converted into active, infectious bacteria.

The C. difficile outbreak at the MTW Trust

Glenn Douglas's arrival as Chief Executive in 2008 coincided with the publication of a report that detailed incredibly high rates of infection at the MTW Trust. Since then, the rates of infection for C. difficile bacteria and MRSA (Methicillin-resistant Staphylococcus aureus) have been greatly reduced. Glenn can now be very proud, as he has transformed the Trust into one of the best performers, in terms of infection rates, in the south-east.

However, back in 2008 the situation was extremely difficult. Glenn describes arriving at MTW and immediately feeling that he was being thrust into the spotlight. This sense of being under intense scrutiny was entirely due to MTW's high rates of hospital-acquired infection and the resulting critical report from the Healthcare Commission. The report stated that 'a substantial number of likely deaths had occurred as a result of infection rates'.

The Healthcare Commission's verdict was widely publicised, and the public lost confidence in the safety of the hospital and in the care offered by its clinicians and other healthcare staff members. Glenn had never witnessed such a loss of confidence in a healthcare facility – people were actually frightened to come into the hospital; drop-in visits plummeted, and pregnant mothers-to-be shunned the Trust.

It wasn't only patients who were dissatisfied. Staff members were also feeling hard done by, since they were taking the brunt of the blame for the infections. Some staff members were in denial about the gravity of the situation, regarding the hospital and the deterioration of its image in the eyes of the public and the mass media. Many front-line Trust staff felt that the management were to blame, but it was ordinary employees who were having to face the full force of negative media coverage and public disapproval.

The full horror of the situation became clear when newspaper reporters began to interview victims of the outbreak and their relatives. One man recalled receiving a phone call from his brother, who had explained that he had been 'sitting in his own diarrhoea and wishing he were dead'. Obviously, the media situation could not have been any worse, and people were loudly decrying a badly broken healthcare system at Maidstone and Tunbridge Wells Trust. One commenter felt that the Trust should simply be 'dissolved'.

From a PR standpoint, the outbreak was disastrous. From a humanitarian point of view, the suffering involved was terrible. Those who died from exposure to the C.

difficile bacterium were tragic victims. Everyone, including the new Chief Executive Glenn Douglas, needed to know how it could have happened.

Over time, Glenn and his colleagues began to put the pieces of the puzzle together, determined to avoid repeating history. The new MTW executive was also determined to rebuild the image of Maidstone and Tunbridge Wells Trust, and to restore confidence – from the public and the media. This was no easy task...

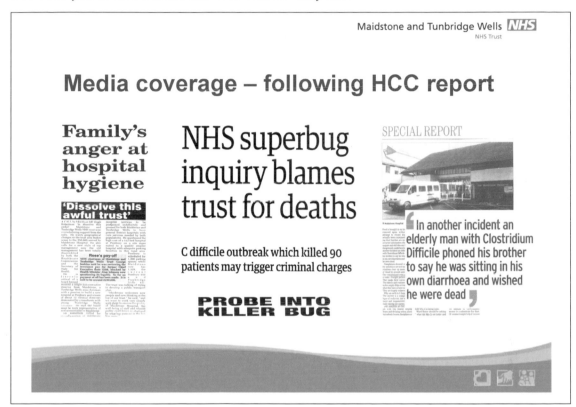

Causes of the outbreak

The causes of the C. difficile outbreak were found to be:

- the lack of nursing staff, both perceived and real
- the fact that cleaning was never given priority within the organisation
- the excessive focus on reducing costs (of course, this was a false economy; the human and financial costs of the outbreak ended up vastly exceeding any savings that may have been achieved by cutting staff, cleaning, etc.)
- poor antibiotic prescribing
- questions over variation in microbiological advice.

53

Many people believed there were significant tensions within the MTW organisation that contributed to the outbreak.

According to Glenn Douglas, there was 'a climate of fear' at MTW. Highly skilled professionals felt unable to contribute to changing processes and rules at the hospital; they also felt that they could not raise any issues with management. Furthermore, patients and visitors were not being listened to, and their opinions were not valued. MTW investigators have since found a great deal of evidence showing that patients, visitors and other groups were trying to raise the alarm about the rise in infection rates long before the outbreak was officially acknowledged. However, these important signals were ignored.

Glenn explains the Trust's perspective in a video that can be viewed on:
www.youtube.com/watch?v = pPlcvdIaEGc&feature = channel&list = UL

Bridging the chasm

Since the outbreak, Glenn and his team at MTW have implemented an open-door policy for interest groups and the media. For example, they invited the well-known investigative BBC television programme *Panorama* into their organisation.

At the time, this caused a lot of controversy among the Trust's directors. However, it was actually a smart move. In time, MTW began to make real progress with moving forward and rebuilding after the outbreak; and Glenn Douglas was certain that the popular *Panorama* television programme would be the right medium to showcase some of the improvements the Trust had achieved.

As a result of his successful attempts to educate the public through the media, Glenn now feels that third-party involvement is very important, especially as the NHS does not generally sell itself as well as it should. In some cases, NHS media teams use complex language that goes over the heads of the audience they are trying to connect with. However, in order to successfully change opinions, a facility's administrators and media team need to explain, in *simple terms*, exactly what has changed, and how the healthcare system has been healed. This is valuable advice that all hospital clinicians and administrators should keep in mind.

In one of Glenn's previous jobs, the entire acute services of one hospital were moved to another hospital. Strangely enough, those most affected by this change were happy with the move (this is rare, to say the least). The key to this unique acceptance of significant change was careful planning. The move was also effectively publicised and rolled out.

During the planning phase, engagement was sought out with as many groups as possible. The issue was discussed with these groups, and most of the groups' members came round to the Trust's point of view, understanding the reasons for moving Acute Care to another facility. Of course, not everyone agreed. But, through the concerted efforts of the Trust's administrators, they came to see why the new structure was important and realised that it was a positive development from a clinical point of view.

In this, and many other similar cases, the change was simply one of location, rather than the actual services provided. From this point of view, Glenn saw the planning phase and group discussions as vital because they gave an opportunity to explain the clinical case for reorganisation of the service.

Rebuilding support

MTW clearly needed to show its honesty as an organisation. People both inside and outside the institution (i.e. staff *and* the general public) had to see that managers were taking steps to improve the service. The facility's reputation as a dishonest establishment had tainted its image, and this needed to change.

Glenn began by renewing engagement with local partners who had previously lost faith in the hospital because of the C. difficile scandal. Friends are vital, especially in the situation MTW was in, and support was imperative. Maidstone and Tunbridge Wells started its own patient involvement group; and this group was used to maintain focus and represent other people within the community. A non-executive director was appointed in a champion role, and she was chosen because of her personal interest in, and experience of, patient engagement.

However, all these efforts would have achieved nothing if the key issues regarding healthcare facility-acquired infection had not been addressed. In the 12 months after the outbreak only three cases of C. difficile were reported in MTW. This is still too high, but it is a very clear sign of improvement.

Conclusion

It is vital that clinicians and staff listen to patients and try to give them what they ask for, in terms of communication and superior healthcare. This is really at the heart of everything. We also need to change staff culture in some healthcare facilities and create the right atmosphere in which feedback is encouraged – from employees to management, and from patients to clinicians.

To put it simply, the C. difficile scandal at Maidstone and Tunbridge Wells could have been avoided if patients, visitors and partners had been listened to. It's so much easier to prevent such tragedies than it is to heal the system after the event.

Chapter 6

Understanding Patient-centred Care

Patient-centred care is a practical and compassionate model that all clinicians should consider adopting. In the patient-centred care model, the patient plays an integral part in decision-making, and is also the focus of all clinician–patient interactions, treatment options and rules governing the way healthcare services are delivered within a national healthcare system.

Views on patient perspective have been provided by Suzie Hughes, Chair of Patient and Carer Network at the Royal College of Physicians. Suzie's contribution to this chapter proved invaluable. The Picker Institute also provided important information.

In the past, the British healthcare system delivered well in terms of clinical care, but fell short when it came to treating patients in a humane fashion. Holistic behaviours and processes were neglected; as a result, patients felt they were being treated like 'numbers', rather than human beings in need of help. The Picker Institute sought to change this, and their ground-breaking work remains a first-rate resource for clinicians wishing to explore the concept of better patient feedback.

The origins of the Picker Institute

The late Harvey Picker, a distinguished American scientist, inventor, manufacturer of X-ray equipment, academic and philanthropist, endowed the Picker-Commonwealth Programme for Patient Centred Care. From this starting point, the Picker Institutes evolved and the first one was founded by Harvey Picker in 1987.

Harvey and his wife Jean (who suffered from a serious recurring illness) had experienced American healthcare, as patients. They realised that the system there was strong on clinical science, but left much to be desired in terms of humanity. They believed that physicians needed to develop the ability to understand the experience of illness as seen 'through the patient's eyes'. They therefore decided to try and persuade the health community to see patient-centred care as a fundamental part of good healthcare – *not* an optional extra for the lucky few.

Initially based at Boston's Beth Israel Hospital and Harvard Medical School, the main thrust of the Picker initiative was to devise new instruments and methods to measure, assess and compare patient experience against eight carefully developed aspects of patient-centred care in a hospital setting.

The idea was that health professionals and healthcare institutions would be encouraged to improve their attitudes towards their patients, as patients' experiences of care were made visible for all to see, and could therefore no longer be ignored.

Picker surveys around the world

Today the Picker Institute in the US is mainly concerned with lobbying for patient-centred care through advocacy, research, support for medical education and special awards. Meanwhile the Picker Institute Europe, an independent charity established in 2001, organises all Picker activities in Europe. This branch carries out a substantial survey programme for the NHS and the private healthcare sector. Under its first Chief Executive, Professor Angela Coulter, the Picker Institute Europe was largely responsible for persuading British policy makers to recognise patient experience as a fundamental element of quality in the NHS.

Currently, under its new Chief Executive, Dr Penny Woods, the task of implementing patient-centred care proceeds apace in Germany, Switzerland, Italy and the United Kingdom.

Picker principles of patient-centred care

Medical investigations and treatments can often be frightening, distressing and painful. It is therefore essential that the quality of care (largely determined by doctors, nurses and managers) should always be exemplary. Healthcare should never become a cause for worry or concern for patients or their relatives. This explains the need for patient-centred care.

The Picker Institute has identified specific issues that are most important to patients. These are:

- Fast access to reliable health advice
- Effective treatment delivered by trusted professionals
- Involvement in decisions and respect for patients' preferences
- Clear, comprehensible information and support for self-care
- Attention to physical and environmental needs
- Emotional support, empathy and respect

- Involvement of, and support for, family and carers
- Continuity of care and smooth transitions.

The Picker Institute Europe

Today the Picker Institute Europe is headed by Chairman Sir Donald Irvine, who is committed to education and policy changes that meet the needs of patients through patient-centred care. Under Irvine's leadership, the Picker Institute Europe is shifting its strategic focus fully onto the implementation of patient-centred care. This is necessary because, while clinical care is generally very good, a minority of doctors and nurses still do not follow patient-centred principles and practices.

How can the Picker Institute Europe help close the gap?

According to Donald Irvine, the Institute can contribute in several valuable ways. (These can be used as a template or simply for inspiration as you plan your own lobbying initiatives or patient-centred care guidelines.) In Sir Donald's own words:

1   We are a key partner for regulators and government in the UK. Recently, we have been developing new surveys for outpatients and maternity service users, and national questions for community health service users.

2   We have successfully developed new ways to support healthcare organisations in acting upon feedback from their service users. For instance:

- We were the first to provide reliable patient surveys for community health services in 2009, by surveying 80 services for eight primary care trusts.

- In the same year, we produced a landmark report on how to measure dignity in the delivery of health and social care.

- Our Frequent Feedback Service provides trusts, individual hospitals, and general practices with 'near real-time' measurements and data, as the basis for quality improvement – this service is being adopted by growing numbers of providers.

- We continue to develop further quality indicators for our clinical partners – these are needed to support their improvement efforts. We believe these indicators should be an integral part of the UK professional revalidation process.

3   We believe that certain basic standards of care should always be achieved. We call these 'always events'. However, the national surveys we co-ordinate show that this is not always the case. For example, in 2008, 18% of inpatients said they did not get the help they needed to eat their meals. And 12% of patients were not told anything about the outcome of their treatment.

We think this situation is unacceptable. While the proportion of patients who do not receive care that meets our standards is not large, the percentages represent significant numbers of patients for whom, in our view, basic standards of care are not fulfilled. To effect further change, we are now working with Picker Incorporated (in the US) to try and find new ways of bringing about the necessary changes.

4   With the Organisation for Economic Co-operation and Development (OECD) we are working to identify and develop a common set of patient experience indicators, which will enable comparison of the performance of healthcare systems internationally.

Looking Ahead

Patient experience is now set to become one of the core measures of healthcare quality in the Western industrialised world. We are proud of the part we have played in bringing this about. Now, implementation is all. Picker Institute Europe is ready and willing to play a full part. Patients should expect no less.

Taking inspiration

As you can see, the work of Irvine and the entire Picker organisation is quite inspirational. It is of course very practical as well. Multi-source feedback is really the only way to guarantee that the thoughts and feelings of patients are being valued.

Using a questionnaire that is similar to the one shown on p. 21 will be an excellent way to mimic the work of the Picker Institute at your own healthcare facility.

According to the GMC, a patient should give feedback about their doctor in the following categories:

- Being polite
- Making you feel at ease
- Listening to you
- Assessing your medical condition
- Explaining your condition and treatment
- Involving you in decisions about your treatment
- Providing or arranging treatment for you

This apparently simple feedback strategy encapsulates the essence of patient-centred care. Doctors who wish to give their patients more attention and *more of a voice* should simply look at the above list and consider what sort of care their service is currently delivering in these crucial areas.

Other characteristics of patient-centred care

The foundation of good patient-centred care is always *respect* – every patient must be treated with the utmost consideration, so that they retain their dignity during the healthcare process. Diagnosis and treatment should be carefully explained, as patients must have detailed information in order to make wise decisions about their own health. Clinicians must value patients, and patients must never feel rushed or degraded in any way as they deal with their health problems and pursue courses of treatment.

Team medicine

The concept of patient-centred healthcare revolves around a compact, integrated team of healthcare professionals who co-ordinate their services to give the patient a more cohesive and holistic care experience. As patients regularly visit different healthcare departments and facilities while undergoing examinations and treatments, it makes sense to adopt a 'team medicine' approach.

This means that all clinicians working with a particular patient will be in contact with each other regarding the patient's health and treatments. This will result in a more organised and interactive healthcare experience, placing the patient at the centre of the healthcare system.

The team medicine concept also works well when it comes to gathering enhanced patient feedback. Small teams can meet to discuss a patient's concerns, and they can make immediate changes that affect the success of their subsequent interactions with that patient. Since issues with clinical care are less common, interpreting feedback on the quality of interactions is really the main priority with patient-centred care.

Enhancing patient-centred care
Provide easy access to information

To augment patient-centred care in hospitals, information services should be added, whether on the Internet, in print or in the form of better signage and/or pamphlets in clinics. For example, in a clinic where many people speak languages other than English, inexpensive pamphlets in other languages may be a useful way to put patients at ease and to explain a little bit about the hospital and its policies and services.

The Internet is an excellent way to build more communication into the patient care experience. Patients will appreciate being able to visit a hospital website and access interactive services from their home computers or mobile phones. Communication and information should be built in to patient care, and then be extended out into the community.

The GMC questionnaire is designed to get feedback from patients. It is returned to the person or organisation running the survey – and a summary of the findings is sent to the clinician. The GMC suggest that this process is carried out approximately every three to five years and probably only requires a sample of about 20 patients each time. They recommend that clinicians give the questionnaire to successive patients at a particular time, rather than giving it to selected patients who they think will give them good feedback!

Multi-Source Feedback: patient questionnaire

4	How good was your doctor today at each of the following? (Please tick one box in each line)	Poor	Less than satisfactory	Satisfactory	Good	Very good	Does not apply
a	Being polite	☐	☐	☐	☐	☐	☐
b	Making you feel at ease	☐	☐	☐	☐	☐	☐
c	Listening to you	☐	☐	☐	☐	☐	☐
d	Assessing your medical condition	☐	☐	☐	☐	☐	☐
e	Explaining your condition and treatment	☐	☐	☐	☐	☐	☐
f	Involving you in decisions about your treatment	☐	☐	☐	☐	☐	☐
g	Providing or arranging treatment for you	☐	☐	☐	☐	☐	☐

General Medical Council

The above questionnaire shows the sort of questions that will be asked in relation to each doctor.

Patient comfort matters

Patient-centred care should be designed to provide optimum comfort for the patient. Aspects that may need attention range from appropriately heated or cooled waiting rooms and examination rooms, to comfortable chairs, pillows, soft hospital gowns ('Johnny shirts' in the USA), current magazines, availability of hot and cold beverages, and so on. Of course, comfort is also an emotional state, so the patient should be put at their ease whenever possible – especially in situations where they will need to endure pain or embarrassment during invasive examinations or procedures. Being touched in intimate places may be difficult for some patients, and experiencing discomfort in front of medical staff may be traumatic or disturbing. Over time, it is all too easy for clinicians to become jaded – or desensitised to the pain or embarrassment that their patients are experiencing. However, for patients these emotions are very raw and all too real. It is therefore vital to show sensitivity to a patient's comfort at every stage of care.

For example, ice-cold speculums or other medical instruments may be extremely uncomfortable or painful for the patient. To understand this from a patient's point of view, consider all aspects of an in-clinic visit – in your experience what makes a patient subtly wince or quietly gasp? These moments obviously indicate discomfort. There may be ways to decrease this – for instance, by warming the instruments or your hands before carrying out an examination – and you should always try to keep any discomfort to a minimum.

However, in cases where discomfort is unavoidable, a simple acknowledgment of the situation, and an expression of empathy, can make the patient feel better about the procedure. Occasionally, doctors become used to small signals that patients are experiencing some degree of discomfort, and they simply ignore these clues, as they are just 'a part of the job'. This is the wrong attitude to take. Everything that happens during an in-clinic session with a patient is very important. After all, these meetings are short, and patients will form opinions about the quality of the healthcare service delivery very quickly. To get the positive feedback you want, you must practise empathy throughout every patient–clinician interaction. In time, this sort of empathy will become the norm, and your patients will feel happier.

Patients who are feeling emotionally uncomfortable during an examination or procedure may become quiet or withdrawn, or (conversely) they may talk too much in order to mask their anxiety. Any sudden changes in demeanour or speech patterns can be very telling, and you should watch out for them during the consultation.

Support networks are vital

Getting the patient's family and close friends involved in their healthcare and self-care can be very beneficial. Effective patient-centred care always recognises and utilises the patient's own support network.

For patients with chronic health conditions – or patients experiencing illnesses that require the assistance of friends and family – support networks can make a huge difference. If a patient would like a family member or friend involved in their at-home care, or in their treatments at the hospital, this request should be honoured as far as possible. Of course, asking the patient whether or not they would like a support group member present during appointments at the clinic should always be a part of good patient-centred care at the outset.

Patients often don't know what is or is not permitted according to hospital rules, so they may be too shy to ask about bringing others to their treatments or examinations. By stepping in and bridging the communication gap, a compassionate clinician can therefore create new channels for patient-centred care that stretch out into the community. Family members and friends will be able to assist the patient in administering self-care; they can also do things that the patient may find difficult during an illness (such as giving medication, making meals, doing housework, bathing the patient, and running errands). Support groups are valuable resources for the patient, offering them information, practical assistance and emotional support. Physicians, nurses and other clinic staff members should therefore hold these groups in high esteem.

Building stronger relationships

Without strong relationships between patients and clinicians, patient-centred care doesn't really work. Nurturing communication and warmth through conversations centred on the patient's particular needs will therefore be very important. As we've learnt, relationships flourish when politeness, concern, good listening and patient comfort are part of the patient–clinician interaction.

However, there are some other factors in building healthy, positive relationships that are likely to lead to better patient outcomes, and these are discussed below.

Infrastructure must support change

In order to build bonds between doctors and patients we need to create a healthcare infrastructure that supports stronger relationships. Our environment has a considerable impact on all of us. Some clinical settings certainly need upgrading, and this may require time and funding. However, in the meantime we all can work on improving our communication skills and sharpening our focus on the patient. This will enable us to achieve better results for patients and better job satisfaction for staff. Once the system is reconfigured, it will be easier for healthcare staff members to learn more about their patients.

Nurses and community healthcare workers must play a role

Nurses and community outreach workers must also do their part to build relationships, since doctors are often stretched very thin, schedule-wise. Nurses provide wonderful services to patients, and they are a prime element in nurturing better relationships between patients and the healthcare system. Community outreach workers and home care nurses may do at-home visits with patients who suffer from chronic illnesses. Obviously, this intimate and personal form of healthcare requires a good level of trust.

Community healthcare workers should therefore devote as much time as possible to getting to know their patients and trying to serve their particular needs. There is more to a person's well-being than treating their medical condition – a more holistic healthcare model will support the well-being of the *whole* person through better relationships. In this way, nurses and community care workers can be powerful forces for change.

How can patients contribute to their own care?

Self-care and monitoring

Self-care and monitoring are important aspects of patient-centred care, and the choices patients make regarding their self-care and monitoring must be respected. However, in some cases patients need to be taught how to carry out this type of self-care and monitoring – and this is where stronger relationships between patients and clinicians play a part.

To gain a patient's trust, and to influence them to make the right choices about their healthcare, a clinician must have a real relationship with the patient. This can be achieved partly through demonstrating respect for the patient's culture, their religion (if any), and their personal preferences. Once a patient senses a physician's respect and concern, that doctor will have more influence with the patient.

Patients as partners

Patient-centred care is all about giving patients more opportunities to make decisions about their own healthcare. The 'patients as partners' concept is also a great way to free clinicians and other healthcare workers from the burden of excessive bureaucracy and red tape.

In the NHS (and other, similar healthcare systems), changes need to be made to fit the 'patients as partners' strategy. This will enable us to measure healthcare outcomes that affect people's lives and well-being, rather than getting bogged down in bureaucratic issues that don't serve the needs of our patients.

When patients become partners in their own healthcare, both staff and patients have more room to think creatively, express themselves, and explore the concept of patient-centred care from the inside. Getting away from the cold and clinical practice of medicine is important – and so is shedding some of the bureaucratic red tape that goes with it.

To employ a 'patients as partners' system, it is vital to redesign the way we measure success. For example, staff must be free to strengthen relationships with patients, without having to account for every second of their time.

Accountability is an issue that must be addressed and defined within the parameters of the new system. Front-line healthcare staff members need to be given enough control to do their jobs properly, while also supporting patient-centred care. From receptionists to nurses to doctors, every staff member must be supported as they adopt better patient feedback methods and learn to interact with patients in a deeper, more caring way.

A shared vision of healthcare

We need to stop measuring everything in terms of time and money. Clinical outcomes are what count in patient-centred care. If treatments are successful, in terms of alleviating disease and suffering and restoring function, patients will be able to work, pay taxes and support their communities. Reducing the numbers of chronic patients will save time and money in any case. There are several ways in which clinicians and administrators can support better clinical outcomes through superior patient–clinician interactions and patient feedback, as discussed below.

Giving patients choices

The idea of sharing treatment choices with a patient may be unfamiliar. Many clinicians are used to having total control over courses of treatment for their patients. However, as so many patients don't stick to treatment suggestions anyway, or never pursue them at all, there is real value in sharing visions for superlative healthcare with patients, and letting them contribute to the decision-making process.

Giving patients choices whenever possible is an excellent way to engage and involve them in their own journey through the NHS (or another similar system). Communicating the pros and cons of various treatment types is at the heart of patient-centred interactions.

Patients must feel knowledgeable, valued, and ready to make choices based on accurate and up-to-date information about their illness and potential treatment options. Doctors must stress communication above all; clinical outcomes will then improve as patients gain new trust in the patient–clinician relationship.

One example of a way to empower patients is by offering them a selection of potential treatments, and letting the patients decide which one would be best for them. But there needs to be some flexibility in this – not every patient will want to make this decision themselves. For instance, some patients may get very anxious if they are told that they have to choose their own hospital or specialist and don't feel equipped to make this decision. Also, not every choice a patient makes will necessarily work out. There will be some trial and error, and some changes to deal with. Patients should be assured that they can change their minds if they feel dissatisfied with their level of care – or with their relationship with a healthcare provider.

Patients should never feel 'locked into a situation'. If they *do* feel trapped, they will be far less likely to continue with the suggested treatment. Care strategies must always be centred on keeping patients happy, so that they will see treatments through and get the full benefit from them. Any rules or processes that stand in the way of giving patients choices should be reassessed and altered.

Some treatments have unpleasant side effects in the short term but it is necessary for the patient to undergo these in order to benefit in the long term. In these situations, clinicians need to take special care to prepare patients for what is to come but also explain the importance of sticking to the treatment in order to get the desired eventual outcome. In the initial discussion about the treatment, patients should be informed about possible side effects and given an opportunity to discuss any concerns they may have. The clinician can recommend strategies and approaches to overcome or reduce the side effects if they occur. (Most possible side effects never actually do occur in the majority of patients.)

Avoid discrimination

Everyone should be allowed to access patient-centred care, which means that no discrimination should ever be permitted. Issues related to sexism, ageism or any other form of discrimination should be dealt with quickly to restore an environment that offers every patient an equal say in their own healthcare treatments and healthcare providers.

People with mental and/or physical disabilities should also have full access to the kind of care they need. For people with disabilities, patient-centred care is extremely important. Often disenfranchised by society, they may need support to get the health-related help they want. It's up to clinicians and healthcare staff to do what is right, and to ensure that every disabled person is allowed to pursue patient-led care to the extent that is appropriate for them.

For example, people with mental health challenges or special needs may require advocates to help them decide on courses of care. In such situations, staff must be committed to working with family, friends, legal guardians or advocates to plan the best course of treatment for the mentally disabled person. Sensitivity, accessibility and accountability must all be stressed during patient-centred care with those who have disabilities.

Every attempt must be made to avoid marginalising any group, including the elderly. The most needy or frail members of society must be protected and given the concern and care they deserve. Anyone practising discrimination against a particular person should be held accountable for their actions.

Doctors may choose to work with local groups that support education and help for those with disabilities. In fact, joining forces with community groups that support people with mental and physical disabilities can be an excellent way to find out what the needs of the disabled really are, and just how they can be supported through patient–clinician interactions and patient-centred care.

Depoliticise healthcare

Ideally, patient-centred care should never be politicised, since this distracts attention from the central aims, which are:

- listening to patients
- giving patients a voice in their own care

- respecting patients' opinions and decisions
- working with community groups to support patients in their local areas
- supporting better self-care techniques and education.

However, in reality there are many ways in which modern healthcare services, such as those provided by the NHS, *are* politicised, to the detriment of patient-centred care. For example, budget overhauls (due to downturns in the world economy or changes in political leadership in a particular country) will inevitably affect healthcare. As governments run national healthcare systems, financial shortfalls and other issues are bound to affect the quality of care delivered to patients – in direct opposition to the ideals of patient-centred care.

Unfortunately, it can be difficult to implement long-term changes that benefit patients when a national election might result in the subsequent dismantling of all the proposed changes. The link between politics and the NHS (or other healthcare systems) is therefore a disadvantage in a sense. However, most politicians from all parties *do* recognise the need for change within the NHS, in view of the dissatisfaction of its end-users, who often feel unheard, unvalued, and rushed through the system.

The current climate of economic austerity is taking its toll on government-funded healthcare systems worldwide – including Britain's National Health Service. In the NHS, healthcare managers are struggling to deal with budget cuts to a system that is already overstretched. The scale of the NHS is vast, with over one million patients being seen every day. Therefore, budget cuts passed down from the political powers-that-be directly affect patient care initiatives in both the short and long term.

This means that there is little investment in expensive new systems for gathering patient feedback and little management time is allocated to discuss implementing organisation-wide systems. Under these circumstances, it is even more important for individual clinical teams and departments to pilot their own approaches to understanding patient experience and improving their team effectiveness. A simple one-page questionnaire can be devised (see example on p. 21) and it will not take much time or money to pilot this.

Breaking through fears and misconceptions

It's widely acknowledged that the way healthcare services are offered to patients directly affects whether or not they choose to utilise them. For example, the perception (or misconception) exists that it's very difficult to see specialists and get the right referrals from a primary care centre. Therefore, many patients who sense that they need specialists and more in-depth care may simply give up on the idea of visiting a primary care institution. When patients feel daunted by the apparent difficulty of getting the care they need, something is wrong, and the issue needs to be addressed. In order to convince patients that they can get a high standard of healthcare via primary care institutions, doctors and administrators must prove that high-quality care and referrals can be easily accessed from these institutions. The problem can therefore partly be solved by strengthening communication between patients and primary care physicians. This improvement should be publicised through media representation that stresses a new era of patient–clinician interaction and patient-led care, using some of the channels listed below.

Media campaigns

Clinicians can act as highly effective advocates for their primary care facilities. In fact, doctors are often excellent media representatives, as long as they've had a little bit of coaching on how to handle questions and which topics they should avoid.

Doctors who wish to reach out and change misconceptions should work with Trust administrators to formulate new strategies, such as interviews on radio or television. The Internet also offers many good opportunities to explain the benefits of patient-centred care, while also clearing up misconceptions regarding the usefulness of primary care.

Blogs

Blogs are a terrific way to reach out on the Internet and educate the general public about the positive aspects of primary care and patient-led care. Blogs written by doctors may be done anonymously or under their own name. The tone should always be positive, politically correct and professional.

Doctors who wish to blog should begin by signing up for a free blogging service, such as the ubiquitous Google's own Blogger service. Once a blog is set up, it's a simple matter to write informative articles about patient-centred care.

Pictures and links may be added to blogs to give them more visual impact and interactivity. In general, blogs should contain fairly short articles of about 400 or 500 words. Some tips for effective blogging (based on the reading patterns of Web 'surfers') are listed below.

Use short paragraphs

This enables you to avoid overwhelming readers – and makes it easy for readers to absorb helpful information in short 'bites'. Most media experts know that short paragraphs are the best way to get a message across to a target audience.

Include images

Plain pages loaded with dense text are anathema to blog readers, who are looking for something lively and visually stimulating. You can please your blog readers (and attract new ones) by choosing fresh, modern images that support and enhance your blog posts and their meaning. There are plenty of royalty-free stock images available – choose a stock image website (such as www.istockphoto.com) and download some no-cost images that are safe to use and share.

Add links

Web links can lead back to Trust or hospital websites, patient associations, support groups and other useful institutions (see, for example, the list on **www.arthritiscentre.org/about-us/useful-links/**). These links offer patients an easy way to learn more about the subject you are addressing. You can also add links to topical articles about patient-centred care. Always test your links after you add them, to check that they work. Links should be carefully chosen to reinforce your overall message.

Articles

Internet 'content farms' are excellent places to spread the word about healthcare advances; they may also offer great opportunities to break down misconceptions about public healthcare systems. To participate in educating the public through content farms, such as Ezine, simply write a 500-word article that fits certain criteria. Generally, these sorts of articles will include:

- an introductory paragraph that presents the topic of the article in layman's terms
- two or three key points, set out in bullet point format; these points, each one in a separate paragraph, will make up the 'body' of your article
- a concluding paragraph that wraps up the topic and re-states your main opinion or idea.

Online videos

The video-sharing website www.youtube.com is hugely popular, and offers an interactive experience to its users, who can leave comments under any user name they wish to adopt. Making an informative video about patient-led healthcare, healthcare misconceptions and other related topics can be a great way to raise public awareness of these important issues. Filming a speech from a professional medical conference or other event can also make a good YouTube video that helps to educate the public. Some examples can be found on the patientinvolvement YouTube channel:

http://www.youtube.com/watch?v = Tj5B1JZONtQ&lr = 1

Personal websites

Many doctors do not have personal websites. However, for those clinicians who wish to engage more with the public-at-large, a personal website can be an interesting idea. Of course, these are not free – first, you will need to choose a domain name and buy that name, and then pay for hosting. Lastly, you may need to pay a website designer or you can purchase a template in order to create good web design and update the site.

There are also some easy-to-use, free templates available such as **http://wordpress.org/**

Podcasts

If you don't mind recording yourself or asking someone else to do it, creating podcasts that you promote on the Internet can be an interesting way to do 'Internet radio' without a big time commitment.

Podcasts are short, recorded conversations or monologues. You may wish to use these to talk about healthcare and the future of patient-centred services. It's easy to promote your podcasts, as well as any other forms of online communication, by posting links to them on other websites, Twitter and Facebook.

Conclusion

As you can see, the concept of patient-centred care is all about giving patients everything they need to be informed, comfortable and valued during the entire patient care cycle. From the first greeting at reception to the final follow-up communication, patient-centred care is designed to make life better for patients while they experience illnesses and health issues.

Better patient feedback methods will support the goals of proper patient-centred care. Surveys, focused patient–clinician interactions, and pre- and post-consultation forms will aid the process and will supply medical teams with the data they need to give patients care that is up to the highest standards and expectations.

To break through fears and misconceptions, doctors and hospital administrators should use both traditional media and the Internet to publicise improvements to the public healthcare system. Creative ways of reaching out to the public will result in better patient feedback.

The ultimate aim of patient-centred care is excellent patient outcomes. Measuring these outcomes is a vital part of examining the way improvements to the healthcare system can better the lives of patients.

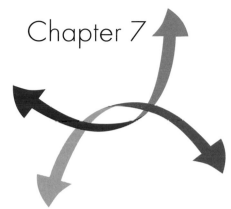

Chapter 7

Achieving Patient Involvement

Achieving patient involvement is a worthy aim but it will not happen overnight. After all, many different people and organisations must come together to bring this goal to fruition. Luckily, leadership and expertise are in plentiful supply within the NHS and other similar national healthcare systems.

Strong leadership can create the right structure for change, and the visionaries who are spearheading greater patient involvement are overseeing a healthcare system that is increasingly inclusive and patient-led. Later in this chapter, I'll share some excellent advice on vision setting in the context of a national health system, much of which comes from the Chief Executive of the NHS, Sir David Nicholson.

Sir Donald Irvine, former GMC President and Chair of the Picker Institute Europe, also offers valuable insights on achieving patient involvement.

Let's begin by exploring some creative and exciting techniques for achieving patient involvement at any healthcare facility. With careful planning and the right attitude, clinicians, administrators and other healthcare staff can come together, working in teams, to create the correct atmosphere for a veritable revolution in patient-centred care.

The best way to spur *involvement* (as opposed to mere engagement) is by making a concerted and consistent effort to connect with patients at their own level. We've already talked about plain speech and its inherent value as it relates to patient–clinician interactions. We've also discussed the many variables that affect the success of an in-clinic visit. We've outlined strategies for building the ideal patient feedback system that enable your team to make small changes that instantly benefit patients.

Throughout the book, general tips on better infrastructure, communication and engagement have provided you with a practical toolkit that should enable you to practise healthcare in a whole new patient-centred way, thus improving clinical outcomes.

This chapter offers further advice that is specifically tailored to promoting meaningful engagement in a host of clinical and community healthcare situations.

Five golden rules of patient involvement

1 Encourage questions

Patients need to feel that they can ask anything that pertains to their health issue, healthcare, and future treatments and prognosis, and there is no such thing as a stupid question. Make sure you tell every patient that you want to hear their questions, and that you are there to answer any queries they have, either during in-clinic appointments, or via phone or email. In our clinic we have a pre-consultation questionnaire to gather information about symptoms. This includes a section telling the patient that they can expect the discussion with the clinician to include:

- diagnosis or possible diagnosis
- prognosis
- further investigations plan
- treatment plan.

If we have not discussed any of these aspects, the patients bring them up for discussion.

2 Get creative about communication

Patients sometimes feel very stressed or upset during medical appointments – their fears or worries about their health may make it difficult for them to take in everything that clinicians say. For this reason, you may want to encourage better communication and patient involvement by telling patients that they are free to record your in-clinic sessions on a Dictaphone or similar device. This way, the patient will have a record of the conversation, and they will be able to replay it when they are feeling less vulnerable, anxious or upset.

Note-taking can also be helpful, but it's not as comprehensive as a recording. Nervous or preoccupied patients are unlikely to take perfect notes.

Finally, the clinical team should send the patient a copy letter relating to the consultation, which is also sent to the other clinicians involved in their care.

3 Ask questions

Asking questions about patients' healthcare preferences, and their perspective on health and treatment approaches, as well as their phobias and dislikes, can forge a stronger bond between patient and doctor. For example, some patients may be terrified of needles or general anaesthesia, but be quite happy to undergo other healthcare procedures such as physiotherapy.

Learning what a patient fears or tolerates easily can be very valuable when planning potential treatment options. It's also a good way to personalise the healthcare delivery system, taking into account individual patient preferences.

Patients often find it helpful to contact a helpline or the nursing team with questions about their treatment. For this reason, it is a good idea to include the contact details of the helpline in each letter they receive.

4 Arrange follow-up appointments

Follow-up appointments can be useful to discuss issues that might encourage more patient involvement. For example, asking patients how they are reacting to a new medication can be useful. Sometimes patients want to talk about side effects and other similar problems, but they fear they may be wasting a busy doctor's time. To make this easier, try to draw them out and spend a little time showing them that you care and are particularly interested in understanding their issues and challenges so they can be addressed.

Studies show that patients may sometimes prefer to discuss certain issues with a nurse rather than a consultant. Where possible, offer patients a choice as to who they see for a follow-up appointment.

5 Encourage self-care

Patients who are unused to practising self-care will need tips, encouragement and the support of healthcare professionals and their friends and family. Getting your patients more involved with self-care through suggestions, follow-up appointments and related treatment options can be an excellent way to form a deeper, more beneficial relationship.

We usually use leaflets and booklets to share information about the condition and treatments for it. These resources inform patients and start them on the journey towards basic self-care. Helpful booklets can usually be obtained from different societies and support groups, and can be adapted for use by individual departments. There are also plenty of software programs available that will help create professional-looking booklets in a very short time – many of these programs can be used for free online. Microsoft Word or Adobe Pagemaker are both good options for this type of project.

Once you have your booklet ready, you can personalise it for the patient by writing their name on top, and giving it to them during the meeting. The patient will be very impressed to get a personalised booklet from a doctor – it shows an extra level of caring, and it will assist the patient in performing safe and beneficial self-care when they are at home. If the patient is elderly and frail or requires a lot of support, make sure their relatives, friends or advocates also have copies of the self-care booklet.

These are just a few examples of how patient involvement can be fostered with the right attitude and behaviour. Any clinician or medical team can utilise these tips to establish trust and rapport with their patients.

The extra work that healthcare teams do to connect with patients and inspire true involvement will require dedication and compassion. However, the benefits derived from these new initiatives will make patients happier as they progress through their treatments. Ultimately, better communication and increased patient feedback will create a win–win situation for both clinician and patient.

Feedback should be efficiently utilised

- The cycle of patient feedback, including a debriefing by a medical team, need only take a few minutes.
- Pre- and post-consultation questionnaires should take less than a minute each for the patients, and post-whole clinic debriefing of the clinical team could be done within 2–5 minutes.
- Issues can be quickly identified and action plans made, sometimes before the next clinic.
- The team should be trained to adhere to regular real-time patient feedback, with team briefing and de-briefing. Many teams that have tried this approach have found it very valuable to combine this with immediate action to resolve any issues.
- Some issues will take longer to resolve or may require support from other departments. For example, there may be issues around patients needing blood tests or resources required to do the clinics in a different way in order to avoid delays in clinical assessment and giving appropriate treatment for urgent medical conditions.

Time management and patient involvement

Improving patient involvement through a strict schedule will ensure that no one is short-changed. This will require a lot of discipline, but it is a very important component in using better patient feedback to ensure positive patient outcomes.

Some useful ways to improve your personal time management are listed below.

1 Allocate blocks of time

Allocate your time in blocks of suitable length, such as 10-minute, 20-minute or 30-minute slots. Clinics can often run late but you should review notes and investigations before the next clinic day and request missing items.

2 Deal with paperwork straight away

I find that dictating a clinic letter immediately after the patient has left is most efficient. Sometimes the dictation may be done with the patient in the room, and this can help summarise the consultation for the patient again. Reviewing the notes and results for the next patient before they come into the consultation room can help you identify any missing information that the team needs to find while the consultation is taking place.

3 Remind your team about time management

All members of the team should be reminded (in the pre-clinic briefing) of the importance of time management. We need to be respectful of patients' time – with everyone working together to keep the clinic running as close to schedule as possible. Of course, there will always be glitches and setbacks. To deal with these issues, you need regular reviews of the challenges. These reviews will enable you to implement small improvements to continually optimise the running of the clinic. For example, if there are delays in pre-clinical weighing, blood pressure and oxygen measurement that hold things up, it may be better to do them after the consultation.

4 End sessions promptly

Sometimes it's very difficult to get a patient to stop talking so that you can end a consultation or other in-clinic session. In general, to avoid this, you should use the first part of your session to address the patient's thoughts and concerns. Then, when examination and treatment options have been explained, ask if the client has 'one or two more questions' and tell them that they will have an opportunity to ask any further questions once they have received the clinic letter and other information. Be polite and set realistic boundaries that keep schedules on track. However, remember that it is important not to rush patients if they clearly have other important concerns that need to be discussed. If necessary, arrange for discussion with another member of the team. If the patient needs to discuss treatment options with their family or review the clinic letter then a return visit could be arranged.

5 Identify the problem areas

If you're struggling with time management, look for patterns and isolate any problems and issues that may need to be addressed. If the issue only arises with certain patients, you may need to approach your relationship with them differently. Structure the next appointment in a new way, and try to control the session throughout, while also allowing time for the patient to express their thoughts and concerns.

6 Be prepared

Being prepared is very important when a new patient feedback system is being rolled out or utilised. You must have your notes ready before the session, including the patient's pre-consultation form. Putting a few simple systems in place will help you to continually improve the running of the clinic by enhancing patient experience and team effectiveness.

Burn-out

Care-givers, such as doctors and nurses (and home carers), are subject to stress and problems that may manifest as burn-out. Burn-out is an issue that should be discussed, as it affects many clinicians, and it does have an impact on the way they relate to patients. Not surprisingly, burnt-out clinicians can sometimes lose their enthusiasm for their work. Dealing with burn-out can be a challenge. However, tackling the issue and dealing with the problem may be an important step in the journey towards better patient involvement.

What is burn-out?

If you're a clinician, you probably already know what burn-out is and what it does to the brain and body. Career-related burn-out usually manifests as feelings of stress, depression and anxiety, in response to the demands of work.

Some doctors are lucky enough to escape burn-out. However, today more than ever, many physicians have become burnt out by the rigours of overscheduling, the emotional demands of the job, and the difficulty of trying to find enough time and space for personal and family life.

The main symptoms of burn-out that may affect relationships with patients include:

- clinical depression
- job dissatisfaction
- exhaustion
- sleep disorders (insomnia is prevalent)
- weight gain or loss
- the feeling of being overwhelmed
- a sense of not being valued by healthcare systems (either at the local or national level).

How to cope with burn-out

In an overburdened public healthcare system, doctors and other healthcare professionals are asked to wear many different hats. Being asked to change their practice and start offering patient-centred care may seem like adding a further burden to the mountain of tasks and responsibilities, thereby contributing to feelings of burn-out.

However, the best antidote to burn-out is for clinicians to be mindful of the reasons why they went into a career in healthcare in the first place. Often, it was because they had a strong sense of vocation and a desire to serve and make a real difference in patients' lives. This is still possible despite the challenges they may be facing.

Here are some tips on coping with/avoiding burn-out.

1 Take regular exercise

Following a healthy exercise regimen is probably something you advise your patients to do on a regular basis – but you must also do it yourself.

Cardio exercise will boost your mood – endorphins will be released, contributing to feelings of pleasure and calm. Of course, if you are a clinician you will understand these things, but depression or burn-out can take away the desire to do what is right for your body.

In order to turn things around, consider buying an exercise cycle or some other home gym equipment that will allow you to get fit without the trouble of going to a gym. Even 30 minutes of vigorous cardio exercise will change the way you feel about life. Problems will feel less burdensome, and your positive attitude will make you more popular with patients.

2 Eat and drink sensibly

Healthcare professionals sometimes find it difficult to eat at regular times or to make choices about the food they eat when they are at work. Although they know the importance of eating small, frequent, nourishing meals and drinking enough water as well as avoiding too many caffeine-containing drinks, they don't always put this knowledge into practice. In some medical training settings, heavy alcohol consumption is common and this can sometimes continue and become an issue in later life. There is evidence that no amount of alcohol is entirely safe – even small amounts can have a negative impact on the neurone connections in the brain.

3 Get support from clinical networks and mentors

Where possible, clinicians and other healthcare professionals should have a network of peers and mentors for mutual support and guidance. When tackling organisational issues (such as lack of admin support, or making the case for getting additional staff or investment in equipment) the experience of colleagues can be very helpful. There is no point in 're-inventing the wheel' and most projects require local and wider support to progress. Help and support can also be offered by confidential helplines, provided by many unions and professional associations.

4 Explore the benefits of therapy

Doctors don't always make the best patients. On the contrary, they may 'shrink' away from being analysed (or metaphorically 'poked and prodded') by anyone. However, clinicians are certainly subject to depression and burn-out. In fact, this segment of the population is statistically proven to be very susceptible to these types of disorders.

Therapy is perhaps more common in the US but that's no reason not to consider making use of it elsewhere. Therapy offers an outlet and a safe place to vent. While it may not always be available through an employer, some physicians prefer to go to a private therapist in their own time (and using their own money). How you choose to get therapy is not really the issue – the issue is recognising that you need it and being willing to do what it takes to get well.

In many ways, it's really quite brave to seek out therapy, and it can be an excellent release when life gets hard. Doctors are expected to be superhuman, but no one is superhuman. You can break the chains of depression and burn-out by seeking a professional therapist who understands what you are going through and how to treat the condition. As you heal others, the right therapist can also heal you.

Burn-out can also affect patients

Patients with chronic health conditions are also subject to burn-out, which may lessen their ability to relate to doctors at in-clinic sessions. Be on the alert for symptoms of burn-out in your patients.

People who are suffering from illnesses may become very stressed or sad – it's only natural to have feelings of tension, fear and melancholy when health problems are a constant issue. However, these feelings can create a barrier that negatively affects the patient–clinician relationship.

By learning more about burn-out, you can spot it more easily in others, and you can treat the whole person, rather than just the chronic illness. If you need to add mental health services to your roster of regular treatments for a patient's disease, by all means make the referral and get the ball rolling (with the patient's agreement). This holistic and humane type of healthcare requires a modern and caring approach to treating the mind, body and spirit – and it really works.

Be careful when questioning a patient about their emotional state, as patients may be sensitive or depressed about their feelings. Society still stigmatises mental illnesses, including depression, although awareness and understanding have increased significantly in recent years.

In general, younger people will be more open about feelings of depression, while older generations may feel that they have to keep a 'stiff upper lip'. This attitude, while commendable in some ways, may lead to inner feelings of despair.

It's really important to look under the surface when interacting with your patients. Try to get to know them in a more meaningful way. Use the psychology of communication to relate to them and observe their verbal and non-verbal cues (see Chapter 4).

Any mental health issues that affect the patient–clinician relationship will cause this relationship to falter. Solving burn-out, whether in yourself or in a patient, can therefore lower the barriers and increase patient involvement.

Get patients interested in being involved

Sometimes, creating an in-hospital media campaign can involve patients – one example might be a mini-campaign about better hand hygiene. A recent study showed that most people's mobile phones carry traces of faecal matter and even E. coli bacteria! Obviously, many people are still not practising proper hand-washing techniques after using the lavatory.

A better hand-washing campaign could be rolled out within the hospital to encourage discussion, education and a higher degree of patient involvement. If the campaign proves successful, it could be shared with the community via interviews, articles and social media.

Such a campaign might include several simple yet effective elements, as described below.

Signs

Attractive signs can be an excellent, low-cost way to grab patients' attention and educate them about important health matters. Improper hand washing leads to the transmission of harmful bacteria that can make people very sick.

Teaching people how to wash their hands properly, for the right amount of time, with the right temperature of water and the right cleansers, can be an excellent way to build self-care practices that benefit all patients.

Signs should be bold and simple, with headlines, taglines, images and a few large-print sentences about proper hand washing. These signs should then be posted in your waiting rooms, examination rooms and general areas of the hospital.

Leaflets

A small leaflet outlining the correct procedure for hand washing could be distributed to patients when they are at in-clinic sessions. Doctors could use the leaflet to make a stronger connection with patients, and to show them that they care about the effects of poor hygiene.

Of course, any self-care topic could be the subject of this type of in-hospital media campaign. Other topics might include tips on taking medication correctly. Many elderly or ill patients must constantly take large doses of different types of medications, and it can be hard for them to keep their dosing schedules organised.

You can help by outlining some strategies for remembering which meds have been taken, and when. People really need this information to stay healthy, and it can contribute to better self-care that will lead to positive patient outcomes.

The top five reasons to work for better patient involvement

1 Improve your public relations

The image of your healthcare facility is significantly affected by word-of-mouth feedback from patients. If your system isn't delivering the services and relationships that people want, *everyone* will hear about it. To improve the image of your Trust or hospital, you should expand your patient-centred care initiatives into the local community.

2 Increase positive feedback

Currently, feedback regarding patient–clinician interactions in the NHS (and other similar national healthcare systems) is not particularly good. This is obviously unsatisfactory for both sides. You can change the face of modern healthcare by changing your patient feedback system. You just need to get organised and collect the data required to make a difference to patients' lives.

3 Further your career prospects

Yes, it may seem a bit self-serving, but doctors who want to shine and sail through the revalidation process must please their patients in order to receive positive feedback from them. Therefore, adopting these principles makes a lot of sense from a career perspective. It is possible to align your ambitions and the desire to be recognised for your work with a patient-centred care model; the two goals do not have to be mutually exclusive. In fact they can positively reinforce each other.

4 Gain better infrastructure

The changes currently taking place within the NHS are altering the infrastructure of the entire organisation. This overhaul is necessary to support patients and to build stronger communication between patients and clinicians. Better infrastructure will also benefit staff, once the transition period is over.

5 Better clinical outcomes

In the end, the most important factors are the success of treatments and the easing of suffering. Every strategy in this book will contribute to better patient outcomes – each step contributes to promoting stronger communication, better self-care and healthier patients.

Healthcare leadership and patient involvement – lessons from Sir David Nicholson

It was a great privilege to have Sir David Nicholson speak at our Royal Society of Medicine Conference (2009), and he offered plenty of insights to all the clinicians and healthcare administrators who attended.

Sir David has written some fascinating articles and papers on improving modern healthcare through proper leadership and better patient involvement. Learning from experts is always highly recommended – especially when they display the dedication and passion for excellence that has defined Sir David Nicholson's tenure as leader of the NHS. With all this in mind, here is some of his advice on making the transition to patient-centred care.

Giving patients control

Having spent decades working at different levels in the NHS, Sir David has learnt that patient-centred care is really about giving patients more control over their own healthcare and decision-making. However, he also knows there is much work still to be done in order to complete the transition to full patient-led healthcare.

He believes that doctors can play a valuable role as guides through the labyrinth of public healthcare. Since doctors have an intimate knowledge of the NHS and how it operates, they should be willing to share this knowledge with their patients, in order to help them navigate the system.

It makes sense to give the patient more knowledge and education, and it will always lead to better patient outcomes. It will also help to justify the huge investment that taxpayers make each year to support the system. When patients aren't happy with their relationships with doctors, the investment by taxpayers may seem like a waste of money. To change the public's attitude toward the NHS, empowering patients is clearly a top priority

According to Sir David, the performance of those local hospitals that are now committed to patient-centred care is extremely good. However, he believes that the way the NHS communicates with the public is still in need of some modernisation. He does understand that the public image of the NHS is important, and the media (as well as healthcare organisations affiliated with the NHS) plays a role in forming people's perceptions of public healthcare.

Sir David has taken steps to move the system towards patient-led care. In his eyes, this transition period has required a lot of courage on the part of NHS staff. After all, these staff members have had to learn how to provide healthcare in a whole new way. Supporting staff members during this sometimes difficult transition phase is one of the key tasks of effective healthcare leaders.

While clinicians must now be more accountable than ever, the type of accountability called for is very different. The old standards of measurement are fading away, and a new era (in which the patient decides what constitutes adequate healthcare) is on the horizon.

Sir David is not opposed to the concept of competition in healthcare. However, he is convinced that any competition between healthcare service deliverers should be based on patient needs. In other words, all competition should be patient-focused and driven by patients themselves.

When patients are offered a choice of clinicians or treatments, they become empowered, and this creates an environment for competition that is beneficial to the patient. The best providers, reinforced by excellent patient feedback and requests for service, will then rise above others and set an example of what modern healthcare should be.

In the past, success in the public healthcare arena was defined by meeting government quotas and targets. However, this method of measuring success is becoming increasingly obsolete. In the new patient care model, success should only be gauged in terms of clinical outcomes that are distinct and impossible to misunderstand. The patient comes first, and bureaucracy exists only to support the quest for better patient outcomes.

These very relevant thoughts and ideas represent the fundamental principles of patient-driven healthcare in the post-millennial age. For modern healthcare administrators, Sir David's hard-won expertise makes him a perfect role model and educator.

The ethics of patient involvement in public healthcare

The policies expressed in the rules and regulations of national healthcare systems, such as the NHS, should morally and ethically support the goal of enhanced patient involvement. Joining with patients or lay representatives to vet policies before they are adopted is the best way to ensure that we have an ethical system that does what it is supposed to do.

The system and its clinicians and healthcare professionals should espouse the principles of transparency, accountability and integrity. Everyone involved with policy-making should be devoted to the same ideal – full patient involvement in every aspect of decision-making that has an impact on the lives of patients.

Healthcare processes, rules and regulations should be regularly reviewed – and guidelines and infrastructure periodically revised to reflect changes that have taken place in hospital settings as a direct result of better patient feedback and improved patient–clinician interactions. Supplementary documentation, including instructions on communicating well with patients and patients' advocacy groups, is also recommended.

Effective and transparent processes are most beneficial to patients. Clear guidelines that make it easier for staff to support patient well-being and better patient outcomes should be valued and upheld. Services that exclude no one based on age, sex, race, or religion should be the gold standard; and these inclusive services should be publicised in the patient community in order to overcome any existing doubts about the fairness of the public healthcare system.

Support for patients should extend beyond the merely clinical. Of course, clinical care is most important, but patients should also get the help they need to deal with psychological issues, disabilities, learning challenges, financial issues, and more. The humane, holistic approach to the practice of medicine is very different from the rushed and somewhat cold approach of previous decades.

Patients must be given all the information they require to make decisions about their healthcare. For example, courses of treatment should be explained in detail, with pros and cons highlighted. Any barriers to patient understanding must be addressed and rectified. Policies to support all these aims are necessary, and lay representatives who are working in the best interests of the public must approve them.

Turning aspirations into reality
A sense of urgency is needed

Patient involvement has real clinical value. The link between patient feedback, patient–doctor interactions and better clinical outcomes is undeniable. Therefore, some urgency is needed when revising the current systems.

Yes, changes do take time to implement; but some changes can be made immediately, and these changes can bring about immediate benefits to patients. Real-time improvements stem from real-time feedback; an effective patient feedback system, as outlined in this book, is a powerful tool for change.

Improving adherence

Improving treatment adherence through increased patient involvement is an idea whose time has come. Many patients suffer from fractures and other painful conditions that might have been avoided if only they had complied with treatment suggestions earlier on. For some reason, these patients did not follow the advice they were given. They have therefore become victims of a healthcare system that, while well intentioned, has not provided them with the support and communication they needed to make healthy choices about their own treatments and self-care.

Better compliance

People should never fall through the cracks when it comes to public healthcare. While some patients will always fail to comply with treatment suggestions, their number is far, far higher at present than it should be. It only takes a glance at some recent articles written about the NHS to ascertain that lack of patient–clinician trust and communication lies at the root of these problems.

In order to boost patient compliance, it is vital that doctors join forces with health organisations to give patients the kind of care they really want. Patients want to feel valued, and for this to happen they need more in-depth conversations and connections with their healthcare providers.

Slowing down healthcare for the greater good

The answer to streamlining NHS cost overruns and patient dissatisfaction in the long run may simply be to … slow down, talk to patients, and find out what they are thinking. The idea of working *for* the patient is clearly the right course of action in a taxpayer-funded public health system.

Better compliance means healthier patients, and anything that can be done to make this goal a reality is to be recommended. Since patient feedback lies at the heart of compliance, improving feedback is clearly the smartest and most compassionate way to bridge the gulf that currently exists between patients and their healthcare system.

'Selling' patient adherence

Now that we've explored the concept of patient involvement, let's look at some related ways of fostering better patient adherence.

The best salespeople know how to pitch ideas, products and concepts to potential customers – convincing and persuading people is their stock in trade. However, doctors who need to convince patients to comply with treatments and self-care often neglect to 'sell' the idea of adherence to their patients.

With patient-centred care, the patient comes first, and giving them the information they need is paramount. However, there is no reason why doctors can't *sell* the value of what they are suggesting while they explain the details to patients. In fact, selling the concept of strict adherence and self-care is really in the patient's best interest.

When successful salespeople sell the problem-solving aspects of a product or service, they also get the client to make an emotional attachment to what they are selling. For example, if you need to ask a patient to perform self-care (such as checking blood sugar) over a certain period of time, they may baulk if you just give them a schedule and ask them to follow it. However, if you explain how following the self-care guidelines will lead to more comfort and better energy, vitality and well-being later on, the patient will be 'hooked'.

Sometimes it's very important to sell services to patients, using a combination of knowledge and subtle salesmanship. Everything you have ever read about selling or marketing products or services can also be applied to 'selling' the benefits of proper treatment adherence for every patient that visits your clinic/healthcare facility.

So the secret of boosting adherence is easy to implement: just tell the patient how it will make their life more pleasant. Don't lie – simply lay out the benefits in a truthful and positive manner.

Conclusion

This chapter has defined what patient involvement is and how it can be achieved. Clearly, there are myriad methods to make the dream of near-perfect patient involvement a reality.

From leadership advice from industry experts, to tips on starting media campaigns in your own hospital or other healthcare facility, there are many exciting ways to refresh and revitalise your clinic's approach to serving the best interests of patients.

Experiment with the different techniques described in this chapter. However, for best results, I would advise you not to alter the model of pre-consultations, in-clinic sessions and post-consultations (followed by a team medicine debriefing). This system is the fundamental root from which better patient involvement grows, and it should always be protected and nurtured.

Chapter 8

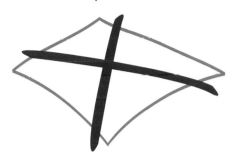

Dealing with Negative Patient Feedback

Negative feedback is very useful when contemplating the improvement of a healthcare system – or *any* type of system. After all, without knowing what is wrong (or what is perceived to be wrong), it is difficult to know exactly how to fix the problem.

However, dealing with negative feedback (which may come in sporadic bursts, or even daily for busy medical practices) is never easy. No one likes to be criticised, and increased patient feedback is bound to lead to plenty of unwanted criticism.

If you're asking patients to tell you what they think, be prepared to hear some unpleasant things. While most patients will be kind and considerate, others may make you feel bad about yourself and the way you practise medicine. In fact, many doctors and other healthcare professionals find the whole process of soliciting and auditing patient feedback very stressful; they would rather avoid the whole process, if possible.

By now, you will realise that patient feedback is definitely necessary. However, this doesn't mean that it's always going to be a pleasant or easy process. To help you cope with processing negative or hurtful remarks, this chapter offers some useful tips on staying strong when handling negativity. If you refer to this advice while implementing your new patient feedback system, you will feel stronger and more capable of persevering through the transition period.

How to handle negative feedback

Anyone who works with the public, or sells a product or service to the public, is going to get some bad reviews. In fact, it's almost unheard of for anyone (whether a clinician, author, actress, chef or entrepreneur) to have an unbroken series of glowing and perfect reviews. Today, bad reviews (as well as good ones) may also pop up on any online message board or social networking site.

You therefore need to know how to handle negative feedback. The first step should always be to look carefully at the feedback and take on board any suggestions and changes you *can* make to improve your effectiveness on the occasion the feedback is based on.

Remember that all feedback is good! In fact, negative feedback is more valuable because it identifies something that happened that could have had a negative impact on the person feeding back, or something that did not run well on that occasion. It therefore provides useful lessons. This is not to say that all feedback is objective and fair but most of the time people do make constructive comments.

Nonetheless, clinicians are of course human beings, with feelings like anyone else. Exposure to too much negative feedback can really hurt. It can actually change the way people (in any profession or at any educational level) view themselves. It's therefore vital to learn some coping mechanisms, as discussed below. These strategies will help preserve self-esteem in the face of wounding criticisms.

Detach from your ego

The wisest people learn to detach from their own egos when they are analysing criticism directed at them. These people are able to see the bigger picture, and they can also understand that this type of criticism is not personal. When looking at (or listening to) feedback from patients, try to remove your ego from the equation, and just focus on what you can do to solve the problem.

Feel your feelings and then move on

Everyone feels bad when they hear negative comments about their own work performance. For clinicians, who generally work very hard to help others, criticism can really sting. Grant yourself permission to feel your feelings and then to get over it. When you've become accustomed to measuring patient feedback more regularly, you will soon learn to take the good with the bad. Regular feedback will reveal the ups and downs that are always part of the transition process.

Set boundaries

While encouraging feedback is healthy, there are some lines that patients should not cross; any profane, sexist or racist insults should be addressed. Setting boundaries is part of getting a new feedback process up and running. In time, your patients will learn what is (and is not) appropriate when leaving feedback. A quiet conversation with a patient who has crossed the line with verbal feedback may be helpful. However, you are not under any obligation to deal with someone who is completely disrespectful or angry.

The GMC cites examples of situations in which the relationship between a clinician and patient may break down – for instance, if the patient has been violent or abusive to you or a colleague, has stolen from the premises or has persistently acted inconsiderately or unreasonably.

They give the following advice:

If you believe there may be scope to restore the professional relationship with your patient, you should make all reasonable efforts to do so. You might find it helpful to discuss the matter with an experienced colleague or your employer/contractor to see whether they can offer any further advice about policies and procedures on ending a professional relationship with a patient before deciding that no more can be done.

In hospital settings, it is rare for patients to be aggressive or abusive. When this does occur, it may arise because of a misunderstanding or because the patient feels they are not being listened to. They may then become frustrated with the situation, rather than with individual clinicians. Showing every patient respect and care when you first greet them may help to calm them down and enable you to discuss any issues they might have. If they have a concern, it is best to deal with it quickly and agree to forward their observation to the appropriate team or person within the institution, so that they can focus on and discuss the clinical issues.

Search for truth

Within many criticisms, there will be elements of truth, which it may sometimes be painful to accept. However, finding the truth and accepting it is extremely beneficial. By facing unpleasant truths and striving to remedy matters, you will become a better clinician and a better person. Some negative comments may be unjustified in certain areas, but hit the nail on the head in others. Your job is to review all the remarks or written comments with an open mind, and do a little self-examination that may lead to a more successful patient–clinician relationship.

Hold on to your ideals

Life is tough, and many people harden as the realities of career and relationships hit home. Criticism can harden people, too. However, there is little value in becoming bitter. In fact, bitterness or hardness just seals you off from your own dreams, goals, emotions and needs. To hold onto your ideals, you have to rise above criticism and see the big picture. Remember that what you are trying to do – in terms of bringing wonderful patient-centred care to your patients – is really important, and it's worth dealing with the occasional negative or derogatory comment along the way in order to achieve this goal.

Connect with patients through feedback

Patient feedback is meant to bring you closer to your patients. You should see it as a bonding exercise because criticism can lead to a better relationship.

Here is the pattern or sequence that leads to a stronger connection.

1 Complaint

The patient makes a complaint or negative comment.

2 Study

The clinician mulls over the criticism and discusses it with their medical team.

3 Action

In the action phase, the clinician makes changes as rapidly as possible, in order to accommodate the needs and wants of the patient (assuming that the patient's request or complaint is logical and contains elements of truth).

4 Connection

On the next follow-up appointment, the patient is made aware of changes that have been made in response to their complaint. If complaints were anonymous, changes to procedure may be posted on a whiteboard in the waiting room area (near the front desk), so that patients can see that suggestions or criticism have been acted upon. As soon as a patient realises that their opinion has been validated, and that their suggestions have been followed, they will feel more valued, and more connected to their clinician.

How to deal with difficult patients

There are some reliable and safe ways to deal with even the most difficult patients – *without* abandoning the principles outlined in this book. Patient-centred care is about inclusion and listening. However, there will always be people who challenge the patience of even the kindest, most compassionate clinicians. For these patients, special tactics and techniques are needed.

Soft-pedal expectations

One tried-and-tested way to deal with difficult patients is by soft-pedalling expectations. Whatever you do, you should never promise a notoriously difficult patient the 'moon and stars' in terms of what you can deliver. The danger of building up expectations with these personality types is that they will tend to lash out when things go even slightly wrong. To give yourself and your team some much-needed leeway, you should be extremely realistic at all times. You will of course want to connect with the patient, but you must also acknowledge the reality of the patient's character and their basic reactions and issues.

Don't argue

With difficult clients, it can be very hard to avoid arguments. One way to avoid these sorts of confrontations is by never directly disagreeing with the patient. Even if you know the patient is making a statement that is wrong, you must carefully consider how to communicate that fact. Telling patients they are wrong is a mistake, as it will only inflame their temper and worsen an already-strained relationship. If a patient hates something or doesn't want to do something, cast about for some practical alternatives. Then give the difficult patient the information they need to choose the right option for themselves. It's a roundabout method, but it does tend to work well in most situations.

Getting a second opinion may be helpful

The other doctors you work with at your healthcare facility can be a source of assistance when things get difficult with a patient. In the new patient-centred care model, it's important to give the patient choices. Therefore, if a patient seems very dissatisfied with your care, despite your best efforts to break down barriers and improve communication, it may be time to refer them to another doctor for a second opinion. Of course, you can do the same for other doctors when they need your help. Building a good relationship with work colleagues can make these situations easier to manage.

Offer extra in-clinic sessions

Another way of pleasing a tough patient is to give them just a touch of preferential treatment. While this is against the rules in theory, it may keep the patient calm until things get resolved to their satisfaction. Offer an extra in-clinic session or two so that you can both clear the air or explore alternative treatments. Always remember that an unhappy, disgruntled patient will probably carry their story of perceived 'mistreatment' (or some other offence) far and wide. It's therefore well worth making maximum effort to satisfy them, even though this can be a bit draining at times.

Always validate the patient's emotions

Patients may lash out or confront doctors because they are feeling frightened, sad or unheard. By asking a patient how they feel and what is bothering them, you may unravel the secrets of their discontent with their treatment. It's entirely possible that a patient is under some form of stress that is contributing to a significant display of unwelcome 'attitude'. By playing psychologist, you may be able to discover whether their emotions are due to medical matters or something else entirely. A difficult patient may be reluctant to 'pour their heart out', but they may be willing to confirm (or hint at) exactly what is making them so irritated at that moment.

Conclusion

Dealing with criticism and difficult patients is part of any healthcare professional's job, but it does take its toll. By practising calming strategies, dealing with animosity wisely, and trying to nip any issues in the bud, you can significantly improve the way you handle stress, conflicts and negative comments.

Of course, there are plenty of other ways to explore handling criticism and other 'hot-button topics'. For example, you could consider visiting a local bookshop to find some self-help books that will teach you how to acquire a calm, Zen mentality. Learning to 'live in the moment' while also seeing the bigger picture is quite a trick, but it can be done.

The Internet is also a powerful resource for doctors who want to polish their personality skills and learn how to handle 'people problems' more effectively. Blogs from industry leaders and experts, along with a huge array of articles and videos, offer many options that may well ease the pressure of making the transition to better patient feedback methods designed to trigger better patient outcomes.

There will always be personality clashes between clinicians and patients. However, when doctors resolve to conduct themselves in a mature, compassionate manner, they can dramatically raise the odds of turning a negative interaction into a positive relationship.

Chapter 9

Measuring Progress

Once a new patient feedback system is up and running, administrators or supervising clinicians must make every effort to use the survey data collected for the greater good. Patient feedback forms (usually anonymous) should be uploaded into a computerised system by a trustworthy data entry typist – one who demonstrates real accuracy and good typing speed.

Every part of a survey should be included in a database. This includes the date, the scores on various segments of the form, and any other unique information, such as extra comments, requests, and so on.

Choose a suitable software package

In general, Excel or Microsoft Project will work well for this purpose. However, any software program that allows for data analysis should work. It's obviously better if everyone is using the same system to update information, so Excel may be a good choice as it is so widely available.

Microsoft Project is a software package that can handle your entire project management needs for a better patient feedback upgrade. MS Project contains a timeline feature, as well as databases, queries, forms and all sorts of analytical tools. It is an excellent piece of software for project managers, but it requires some training, and most staff members aren't likely to be using it regularly.

Measuring clinical outcomes

Florence Nightingale was one of the pioneers of measuring clinical outcomes. By collecting and analysing raw data after she had treated soldiers in the Crimean War, she found weaknesses in the system of diagnosis, treatment and follow-up, and proceeded to revise the system for better efficacy.

The science of measuring clinical outcomes has come a long way since the nineteenth century but the principles remain the same. Nowadays, there are also plenty of questions to be answered regarding exactly which analysis methods will be most valuable to the future of patient-led care.

Knowing the patient

Spreadsheets, formulae and hard numbers or scales of measurement can be invaluable. However, there is another element to the best clinical outcome measurements that is harder to quantify but no less important. *Knowing the patient* is absolutely vital – in fact, lapses in this particular area have damaged the reputation of the NHS, which is currently changing many of its methods and processes to inspire better doctor–patient relationships.

Essentially, without knowing the person and how they think, act and feel, it is impossible to know if their treatment is successful in their own eyes. Of course, some clinical outcomes will be obvious – successful cancer treatments are one example. However, other healthcare issues will not have such hard-and-fast 'good or bad' results.

For this 'grey area', the patient's own thoughts and feelings are the ultimate expression of the clinical outcome. It's therefore very important to follow through on feedback throughout the entire patient care experience. Working with community organisations that support self-care for patients with chronic illnesses is also a great way to stay in touch with patients and see how they are faring in the long term.

The point is – it's all about the patient and how they are feeling. Are they feeling better – or worse? How did their patient care experience colour their view of the public healthcare system? Were they happy with the way things went?

Questions like these are vital components in deciphering the greyer areas of clinical outcomes. For planning purposes, spreadsheets and other such tools are useful resources that help us to identify overall patterns. For humane, holistic purposes, knowing the individual patient is all-important. The point of the exercise is to make each patient happy, as far as possible, in the light of their healthcare challenges.

In the past, success in public healthcare was measured very differently. The system became too bureaucratic and too corporate, and the patients were somehow forgotten in the quest to follow guidelines and meet targets. The NHS and other similar healthcare systems have learnt from the mistakes of the past – they are forging ahead with patient-led care that is all about communication, compassion and clinical outcomes.

Randomised, controlled trials are not enough

The randomised, controlled trials of the past gave us glimpses into the patient care experience. However, these types of measurement were simply not comprehensive enough. Like random drug testing for Olympic or Tour de France athletes, the results did not show the whole truth; they only showed part of the truth.

To take care of patients and to value them properly, as they deserve, every patient must therefore be monitored to the best of the system's ability. With the patient feedback system outlined in this book, no one falls through the cracks. When all the patients' voices come together in unison, we will hear a chorus that truly reflects the current state of modern healthcare. Until that time, we need to build on patient-led care and better patient feedback methods.

Data security

Measuring clinical outcomes from patient feedback forms must always be done carefully. There should never be any loss of data, or any breach of doctor–patient confidentiality. While anonymous patient feedback forms contain a primary level of protection, there are still ways in which the system can be abused.

Protecting the privacy of patients should be a priority during the planning phase and the roll-out of any new patient feedback system. The way data is stored, uploaded and analysed should also protect the privacy of clients, who rely on the public healthcare system's commitment to honouring its confidentiality agreement with patients.

A medical team or committee composed of hospital administrators and clinicians should meet to establish security guidelines and other rules for managing paper forms and uploads of patient feedback. This meeting should occur before any patient feedback forms are collected.

Today, there are many excellent ways to guard data – even modern cloud computing software can be used to add layers of protection to a computer system. Of course, all the usual anti-malware, anti-spyware and anti-virus programs should also be used in any situation where data may be accessed by hackers or other cyber-criminals.

It's a sad fact that some healthcare workers breach the honour code (and the law) by accessing records and feedback that they have no right to see. It is therefore very important to limit the chain of command and keep a tight rein on private information. The strictest possible controls on data security and the privacy and security of files and forms (even anonymous forms) must always be observed. After all, even anonymous forms may contain identifying information, in the form of extended comments that personalise the form.

Staff should be trained in how to deal with paperwork and computer files. Only those who need to see the forms should have access to them, and security processes should be audited regularly to check for any breaches that might have an impact on patient privacy. These issues may seem daunting, but they can be dealt with easily by having an organised approach. Planning processes and methods of measurement for patient feedback will result in a consistent effort that helps to improve patient care experiences.

It is wise to get legal advice regarding any disclaimers or waivers that may need to be signed by patients or added to patient feedback forms. Putting all this in place at the outset can help you avoid a lot of headaches later on, and it will assist medical teams in getting the system up and running.

Patients' needs are not being met at present – so these changes should be implemented immediately. Urgency and a sense of mission should combine with practical concerns and doctors should never lose sight of the bigger picture.

Conclusion

My career as a clinician has blessed me with all manner of positive relationships, including important connections with my patients, incredible colleagues and generous mentors. Working with a diverse range of organisations and people has given me the insights that I have sought to share in this book, in an attempt to improve patient outcomes and team effectiveness.

I believe in the future of national healthcare, and I know that better patient feedback is at the root of positive clinical outcomes. By identifying weaknesses in the system, consulting with experts, and formulating successful patient feedback methods, I've done my best to supply clinicians with the data they need to make a difference to their patients' lives.

This type of patient feedback system will work in any clinical setting – all it takes is the discipline to follow through for each and every patient. Clinicians must devote themselves to better communication and patient-led consultations. Empowering the patient is vital, and putting a more humane face on healthcare services is clearly the way forward.

Over time, the benefits of enhanced patient feedback will become apparent, and patients will begin to regain their trust in public healthcare. Relationships between patients and clinicians will thrive as the entire healthcare paradigm shifts.

To give your patients the best, put them first, and use their feedback to keep building improvements into the healthcare system. With this book, you will have what you need to change the face of modern healthcare delivery, and your patients will feel valued, cared for, and heard.

Index